Contributors

Members of the Renal Standards and Audit Sub-Committee

All are consultant nephrologists unless otherwise stated

Alison M MacLeod (Chair), Professor in Medicine and Therapeutics, Honorary consultant nephrologist, University of Aberdeen, Foresterhill, Aberdeen

Mark T Bevan Lecturer in Nursing, School of Health Care Studies, University of Leeds

J Stewart Cameron Emeritus Professor of Nephrology, Guy's Hospital, London

Gerald A Coles University of Wales College of Medicine, Cardiff

Andrew Davenport Department of Nephrology and Transplantation, Royal Free Hospital, London

Simon J Davies Department of Nephrology, North Staffordshire Hospital, Stoke on Trent

Terry Feest Chairman, UK Renal Registry, and Department of Renal Medicine, Southmead Hospital, Bristol

John Firth Department of Renal Medicine, Addenbrookes Hospital, Cambridge

Ram Gokal Department of Renal Medicine, Manchester Royal Infirmary

Timothy Goodship Reader in Nephrology, Honorary consultant nephrologist, Renal Unit, Royal Victoria Infirmary, Newcastle-upon-Tyne; Secretary, Renal Association (1997–2001)

Peter Gower Renal Unit, Charing Cross Hospital, London

Roger N Greenwood Renal Unit, Lister Hospital, East and North Herts NHS Trust, Stevenage; Vice Chairman, Kidney Alliance

Nicholas A Hoenich Clinical Scientist, Department of Nephrology, School of Clinical Medical Sciences, Medical School, University of Newcastle

Anthony J Nicholls Renal Unit, Royal Devon and Exeter Hospital, Exeter

Stephen H Powis Moorhead Professor of Renal Medicine and Centre Director, Centre for Nephrology, Royal Free and University College Medical School, Royal Free Campus, London

Andrew J Rees Regius Professor of Medicine, Honorary consultant nephrologist, University of Aberdeen; President, Renal Association

Lesley Rees Renal Unit, Great Ormond Street Hospital NHS Trust, London; Secretary, British Association of Paediatric Nephrology

Paul Roderick Senior Lecturer in Public Health Medicine, Wessex Institute for Health Research and Development, Level B, South Academic Block, Southampton General Hospital

R Stuart C Rodger Renal Unit, Western Infirmary, Glasgow

Val Said Kidney Patients' Association, National Kidney Federation

Alasdair Short Consultant in Intensive Care Medicine, Broomfield Hospital, Chelmsford (Intensive Care Society)

Charles RV Tomson Department of Renal Medicine, Southmead Hospital, Bristol

Robert Wilkinson Professor of Renal Medicine, RCIU, Freeman Hospital, Newcastle-upon-Tyne; Chairman, Royal College of Physicians Joint Specialty Committee (1997–2000)

continued

Gwyn Williams Professor of Medicine, Honorary consultant nephrologist, Guy's Hospital, London; President, Renal Association (1998–2000)

Adrian S Woolf Nephro-Urology Unit, Institute of Child Health, London; Secretary, Renal Association

Observers

Jane Verity Leader, Renal Policy Team, Department of Health, Wellington House, 135 Waterloo Road, London

Aileen Keel Deputy Chief Medical Officer, Department of Health, Scottish NHS Management Executive, Scottish Office, St Andrews House, Edinburgh

Philip McClements Principal Medical Officer, Health & Social Services Executive, Dundonald House, Upper Newtownards Road, Belfast

Cathy White National Assembly for Wales, Health & Well Being Strategy & Planning Team 2, 4th Floor Government Offices, Cathays Park, Cardiff

James Barbour Chief Executive, Lothian Health Board, Deaconess House, 148 Pleasance, Edinburgh

Co-authors

Those who were not on the Standards Sub-committee who co-authored sections of the document. All co-authors are consultant nephrologists unless otherwise stated.

Mark G Bradbury Royal Manchester Children's Hospital, Pendlebury, Manchester

J Andrew Bradley Professor of Surgery, Addensbrooks Hospital, Cambridge (President, British Transplantation Society)

J Douglas Briggs Renal Unit, Western Infirmary, Glasgow

Nicholas Fluck Renal Unit, Aberdeen Royal Infirmary

Robert Foley Renal Unit, Hope Hospital, Salford

John L R Forsyth Consultant Surgeon, Transplantation Unit, Royal Infirmary, Edinburgh (Secretary, British Transplantation Society)

Andrea W Harmer Consultant Clinical Scientist, National Blood Service, Sheffield

Alan G Jardine Senior Lecturer, University of Glasgow; Department of Medicine and Therapeutics, Gardiner Institute, Glasgow

Izhar Khan Renal Unit, Aberdeen Royal Infirmary

David Milford Department of Nephrology, Birmingham Children's Hospital

Robert J Postlethwaite Royal Manchester Children's Hospital, Pendlebury, Manchester

E Jane Tizard Renal Unit, Bristol Royal Hospital for Children

Alan Watson Children & Young People's Kidney Unit, Nottingham City Hospital NHS Trust

Nicholas JA Webb Royal Manchester Children's Hospital, Pendlebury, Manchester

THE RENAL ASSOCIATION

Treatment of adults and children with renal failure

Standards and audit measures

THIRD EDITION

Prepared by the Standards and Audit Subcommittee of the Renal Association on behalf of
the RENAL ASSOCIATION and the ROYAL COLLEGE OF PHYSICIANS OF LONDON
in collaboration with the BRITISH TRANSPLANTATION SOCIETY, the INTENSIVE CARE SOCIETY
and the BRITISH ASSOCIATION OF PAEDIATRIC NEPHROLOGISTS

AUGUST 2002

Royal College of Physicians of London
11 St Andrews Place, Regent's Park, London NW1 4LE

Registered Charity No 210508

Copyright © 2002 Royal College of Physicians of London and the Renal Association

ISBN 1 86016 105 7

Typeset by Dan-Set Graphics, Telford, Shropshire
Printed in Great Britain by The Lavenham Press Ltd, Sudbury, Suffolk

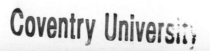

Chapters and authors

The recommendations and standards set out in this publication are based on graded evidence backed by a broad consensus opinion of those who participated in formulating them. Those who drafted and revised the chapters following discussions are listed below.

Foreword

It is a pleasure to welcome the third edition of the Renal Association and Royal College of Physicians' Standards Document *Treatments of adults and children with renal failure*. The 'standards document' has become such an accepted part of British nephrology that it is difficult to remember how radical the first edition appeared when it was published in 1995. It is also remarkable how small the evidence base was at that time. Indeed the first edition was in reality a consensus statement, a mere 26 pages in length. Nevertheless, it provided the framework for the 1997 edition, which capitalised on the new data available from the emerging discipline of evidence-based medicine. The third edition continues the approach and its conclusions are based on a more rigorous analysis of all the evidence available. The resulting document demonstrates how swiftly the evidence base is enlarging. However, it needs to be recognised that insufficient data are available in many important clinical areas, which emphasises the need for yet more work.

The third edition is not just an updated version but contains other important changes. We are delighted that it now includes a fully integrated set of standards for the treatment of children with renal failure. This has been made possible through a partnership between the Renal Association and the British Association of Paediatric Nephrologists. Each chapter now contains a separate section on standards for the care for children, rather than an appendix describing special arrangements for children that was found in the last edition. We are also grateful for our collaborations with the British Transplantation Society and the Intensive Care Society that have enabled us to produce uniform standards in the areas of mutual concern. Some of the standards have already been adopted by the Clinical Standards Board in Scotland and we believe they will be of equal value to those currently developing the Renal National Service Framework. The document has the support of the Royal College of Paediatrics and Child Health, and the Royal Colleges of Physicians of Edinburgh and Glasgow.

The task of compiling this document has been the responsibility of the Renal Association's Standards & Audit Subcommittee chaired by Professor Alison MacLeod. Their enormous collective and individual contributions should be acknowledged. Individual committee members were assigned to lead the reviews of evidence in different areas and draft the relevant chapter prior to discussion at committee meetings. Lastly, we are also especially grateful to the staff of the Royal College of Physicians' publications unit for completing this mammoth task. It is our intention that the document will have the widest possible circulation to inform all those providing renal services of which we can justifiably be proud.

Andrew J Rees
President, Renal Association

Carol Black
President, Royal College of Physicians of London

Contents

1 | Methods of guideline development

2 | Epidemiology of chronic renal failure and renal replacement therapy

3 | Haemodialysis – clinical standards and targets

4 | Peritoneal dialysis

5 | Haemodialysis and peritoneal dialysis: nutritional and biochemical standards

6 | Cardiovascular risk factors in patients on dialysis

7 | Anaemia in patients with chronic renal failure

8 | Transplantation

Introduction

In 1995 the Renal Association produced the first edition of this document which was a consensus statement of recommended standards and good practice for the treatment of renal failure.[1] It complemented the Association's other document, *Provision of services for adult patients with renal disease in the United Kingdom*[2] which described the resources required for service delivery. A second edition was produced in 1997[3] and included chapters on transplantation, acute renal failure and a paediatric addendum. In this third edition we have again produced chapters jointly with the British Transplantation Society and the Intensive Care Society on transplantation and acute renal failure. In addition, a paediatric section to each chapter has been written in conjunction with the British Association of Paediatric Nephrology. Furthermore there are now separate chapters on nutrition and biochemistry in end stage renal disease and anaemia in chronic renal failure; there is also a new chapter on the management of cardiovascular risk factors. For non-specialist readers we have again included a section on clinical aspects of renal failure in non-technical language (Appendix B) and have added a glossary and list of abbreviations used (Appendix C). The standards and recommendations are summarised on the dark edged pages at the front of the document.

How the standards are implemented in individual renal units will depend upon local circumstances and, as indicated in the last edition, units should, after discussion, develop an agreed system of written protocols upon which practice in the unit should be based. In addition all units should submit data to the UK Renal Registry in Bristol or the Scottish Renal Registry in Glasgow so that achievement of standards nationally can be monitored. The number of units submitting data to the registries has increased considerably since the last edition of this document and work is currently underway to record patients' coexisting illnesses so that ability to achieve the standards can be adjusted for comorbidity.

There is concern nationally that outcomes for patients with end stage renal disease are worse in the UK than in other European countries[4] as they are for some cancers[5] and heart disease.[6] We know that the UK spends only 6.9% of gross domestic product on health compared with 9.4% in France and 8.7% in the Netherlands (OECD Health Data 2001). In 2001 the Minister for Health said that the government recognised 'the difficulties for kidney patients and the inadequate service they have endured as a result of decades of neglect and under investment'. Work on a National Service Framework (NSF) for Renal Services is under way with the aim of optimising service delivery for patients with renal failure. This standards document and the NSF are therefore complementary with the clinical standards informing the discussion on service standards in the NSF. These initiatives along with the government's promised increase in spending on the NHS[7] should lead to improved care for people with renal failure.

References

1   Renal Association standards subcommittee. *Treatment of adult patients with renal failure: recommended standards and audit measures* (1st edition). London: Royal College of Physicians, 1995.

2   Renal Association. Working group of the Renal Association subcommittee on provision of treatment for chronic renal failure. *Provision of services for adult patients with renal disease in the United Kingdom*. London: Royal College of Physicians and the Renal Association, 1991.

3   Renal Association Standards and Audit Subcommittee. *Treatment of adult patients with renal failure: recommended standards and audit measures* (2nd edition). London: Royal College of Physicians, 1997.

4   Khan IH, Campbell M, Cantarovich D *et al*. Survival on renal replacement therapy in Europe: is there a centre effect? *Nephrology Dialysis Transplantation* 1996; **11**: 300-7.

5   Berrino F, Gatta G, Chessa E *et al*. Introduction: The Eurocare II study. *European Journal of Cancer* 1998; **34**: 2139-53.

6   Law M, Wald N. Why heart disease mortality is low in France: the time log explanation. *Br Med J* 1999; **318**: 1471-80.

7   Robinson R. Gold for the NHS. *Br Med J* 2002; **324**:987–8.

Acknowledgements

I should like to thank the chapter authors for their considerable efforts in producing and revising the various chapters and all the members of the sub-committee for their comments and help in shaping the document. The renal community throughout the UK made many helpful comments by email or letter, which were very much appreciated. I am grateful to the representatives of the UK Department of Health who have observed the process of development of this document and made valuable suggestions about its content.
Special thanks are owed to Ms Val Said for representing the National Federation of Kidney Patients' Association, and to Dr Charlie Tomson for executing the arduous role of secretary to the sub-committee so successfully. Without the secretarial assistance of Ms Carol Ritchie, Ms Jane Edwards and, particularly, Mrs June Roxburgh, this document could not have been produced. I am very grateful to them all for their hard work and to June for her patience throughout the production of the document. I should like to acknowledge the skilful help of the staff in the College Publications unit and the Presidents and Executive of the Renal Association for their support throughout this endeavour.

Alison M MacLeod
Chair, Standards and Audit Subcommittee of the Renal Association

Summary of standards

2 Epidemiology of chronic renal failure and renal replacement therapy

What is the level of population need for renal replacement therapy ?

Standards

▶ While it is difficult to be precise about the level of national need for renal replacement therapy (RRT), a realistic figure is an acceptance rate of at least 120–130 pmp. **(B)**

▶ It is likely that a minimum level of 100 pmp would apply to all health authorities/boards. **(B)**

Measuring RRT rates

Standard

▶ The Renal Registry definition of acceptance should be used in all units. **(C)**

Recommendation

▶ Each health authority/health board should assess its likely need for RRT in the light of the characteristics of the local population. These rates should be age and sex standardised and in future be standardised for ethnic minority populations, using 2002 Census data on health authority ethnic composition and Registry data on ethnicity. Such recording should be encouraged. **(Good statistical practice)**

90-day rule

Recommendation

▶ To allow meaningful comparison, UK performance should be analysed not only from the day of starting uninterrupted dialysis (day 0) but also from day 90. **(Good statistical practice)**

Late referral

Recommendations

▶ All renal units should audit late referrals to identify avoidable factors and any scope for improving the interface between primary and secondary care providers. **(Good practice)**

▶ Data should be provided to the Renal Registry on date of first referral to the renal unit, and unplanned dialysis, so that the national pattern of late referral and its variation can be established. **(Good epidemiological practice)**

Analysing survival on RRT

Recommendations

▶ All units registered with the Registry should endeavour to supply co-morbidity data on newly accepted patients. The priority should be diabetes as a cause of end stage renal disease (ESRD) and evidence of coronary heart disease or peripheral vascular disease. (**Good practice**)

▶ Survival analyses must at least take account of age, gender, diabetes and co-morbidity. (**C**)

▶ The Karnofsky performance status is a simple measure that could be collected on incident and prevalent patients and used in survival analyses. (**B**)

3 Haemodialysis – clinical standards and targets

Dialysis equipment and disposables*

Standards

▶ All equipment used in the delivery and monitoring of therapy should comply with the relevant Standards for medical electrical equipment (BS-EN 60601-2-16: 1998, BS5724-2-16:1998. Medical electrical equipment. Particular requirements for safety. Particular requirements for the safety of haemodialysis (HD), haemodiafiltration and haemofiltration equipment). (**Good practice**)

▶ Disposables such as dialysers and associated devices are classified as medical devices and should display the CE mark. The presence of such a mark signifies compliance with the national and interntional standards: haemodialysers, haemodiafilters, haemofilters, haemoconcentrators and their extra corporeal circuits (BS-EN 1283: 1996). Plasma filters (BS/150 13960).

Recommendation

▶ Machines should be considered for replacement after seven years' service or after completing 50,000 hours operation, whichever is first. (**Good practice**)

Concentrates and water for dialysis

Standards

▶ Concentrates used, either purchased ready-made or manufactured 'in house' must meet the requirements of prEN 13867: 2002 (concentrates for HD and related therapies). (**Good practice**)

▶ Water used in preparation of dialysis fluid must meet the requirements of BS ISO 13959 2001 (water for HD and related therapies) for bacterial and chemical contaminants. If routine monitoring demonstrates continuous excess contamination, a phased programme to improve this should ensue. When alternatives to conventional HD with low flux membranes are used, such as haemodiafiltration and haemofiltration, more stringent limits in respect of bacterial contamination are mandatory. For such alternative applications microbial count should not exceed 0 Colony Forming Units (CFU)/ml and endotoxin level should be less than .015 IU/ml. (**Good practice**)

*See appendix D for details of standards abbreviations used in this chapter.

▶ A routine testing procedure for product and feed water should form part of the renal unit policy. Samples should be cultured on Tryptone Glucose Extract Agar or Reasoner's 2A and, for fungi and yeast, on malt extract agar or Sabourad's Dextrose Agar, (all incubations at room temperature, ie 20–22°C). The frequency for testing should not fall below monthly and should be sufficiently frequent to detect trends. (**Good practice**)

Dialysate

Standard

▶ The dialysate should contain bicarbonate as the buffer. (**A**)

Dialysis membranes

Standards

▶ Patients whose estimated life expectancy is more than seven years and who are unlikely to receive a transplant as a result of human major histocompatibility complex (HLA) sensitisation, high risk of recurrent disease, rare tissue type or other contra-indications (including personal choice), are at high risk of dialysis-related amyloidosis. Such patients, and those with symptoms of dialysis-related amyloidosis should, where possible, receive a dialysis regimen with better clearance of beta 2–microglobulin, and ultrapure dialysate. Such treatments include HD with high flux synthetic membranes and haemodiafiltration. (**B**)

▶ For other patients the balance of evidence favours the use of low flux synthetic and modified cellulose membranes over unmodified cellulose membranes. (**A**)

▶ Those reusing dialysers marked 'for single use only' should have read MDA Device Bulletin DB 2000(04) *Single-use medical devices: implications and consequences of reuse*. (**Good practice**)

Dialysis frequency and dose

Standards

▶ HD should take place at least three times per week in nearly all patients. Reduction of dialysis frequency to twice per week because of insufficient dialysis facilities is unacceptable. (**Good practice**)

▶ Every patient receiving thrice weekly HD should show:
either   urea reduction ratio (URR) consistently >65%
or   equilibrated *Kt/V* of >1.2 (calculated from pre- and post-dialysis urea values, duration of dialysis and weight loss during dialysis). (**B**)

Recommendations

▶ Patients receiving twice weekly dialysis for reasons of geography should receive a higher sessional dose of dialysis, with a total *Kt/V* urea (combined residual renal and HD) of >1.8. If this cannot be achieved, then it should be recognised that there is a compromise between the practicalities of dialysis and the patient's long-term health. (**Good practice**)

▶ Measurement of the 'dose' or 'adequacy' of HD should be performed monthly in all patients. All dialysis units should collect, and report to the Registry, data on pre- and post-dialysis urea values, duration of dialysis, and weight loss during dialysis. (**Good practice**)

continued

▶ Post-dialysis blood samples should be collected either by the slow-flow method, the simplified stop-flow method, or the stop-dialysate-flow method (Appendix 2). The method used should remain consistent within renal units and should be reported to the Registry. **(B)**

Dialysis-related hypotension

Recommendation

▶ Data on the frequency of dialysis-related hypotension, defined as an acute symptomatic fall in blood pressure during dialysis requiring immediate intervention to prevent syncope, should be collected and reported to the Renal Registry. **(Good practice)**

Vascular access

Recommendations

▶ At least 67% of patients presenting within three months of dialysis should start HD with a usable native arteriovenous fistula. **(Good practice)**

▶ At least 80% of prevalent HD patients should be dialysed using a native arteriovenous fistula. **(Good practice)**

▶ No patient already requiring dialysis should wait more than four weeks for fistula construction including those who present late. **(Good practice)**

▶ All dialysis units should collect data on infections related to dialysis catheters and polytetrafluoroethylene (PTFE) grafts to allow internal audit. **(Good practice)**

Paediatric section

The dialysis centre

Standard

▶ All children requiring HD should be treated in a designated paediatric nephrology and dialysis centre. **(Good practice)**

Recommendations

▶ Children and parents should be free to choose a particular dialysis modality in discussion with the multi-professional team. **(Good practice)**

▶ It is essential that children receiving chronic HD treatment are given a service that meets their physical and psychosocial needs. Children should be nursed in paediatric units where a renally trained children's nurse is always available for advice and support. **(Good practice)**

▶ The child and family should be prepared either in hospital or at home for HD by their named nurse and play specialist using such materials as dolls, videos, story books and games. **(Good practice)**

▶ The child's nutritional status should be managed and monitored by a paediatric renal dietician. **(Good practice)**

Vascular access

▶ Temporary central venous lines risk the loss of potential access points and their use should be kept to a minimum. (**Good practice**)

▶ When tunnelled, cuffed central venous catheters are used, the rate of infection should be better than one in every 12 patient months averaged over the total population for three years. (**Good practice**)

Recommendations

▶ The choice of vascular access should take into account the age and size of the child. Although an arteriovenous fistula is regarded as the best long-term vascular access, this may not be possible in small children who can be managed using catheters that are tunnelled subcutaneously. Such catheters can also provide vascular access in older children where early transplantation is anticipated. (**Good practice**)

▶ Vascular access should be performed by an appropriately trained surgeon. (**Good practice**)

▶ Problems with needle phobia require referral to a child psychologist. (**Good practice**)

Dialysis frequency and dose

Standards

▶ Standards of adequacy recommended for adult patients should be regarded as the minimum for children. (**Good practice**)

▶ Adequacy tests should be performed monthly. (**Good practice**)

Psychosocial support (for HD and peritoneal dialysis)

Standard

▶ Psychosocial support is an essential part of the care offered to children and families while on dialysis. All members of the multidisciplinary team contribute to such support, but the social worker and psychologist will play lead roles. (**Good practice**)

Recommendations

▶ Each paediatric unit should have a suitably qualified and experienced social worker allocated to the work of the unit and involved in arranging appropriate information and support for each family. In addition, the social worker should assess the economic impact of dialysis on the family and discuss possible sources of financial support. (**Good practice**)

▶ Dialysis, particularly in infants, imposes a large burden of care upon families. Strategies such as home-care nursing, respite care and holidays for children need to be considered to prevent family burn-out. (**Good practice**)

▶ Children attending the HD unit on a regular basis have the greatest need for educational support as they will miss considerable school time. Liaison between the hospital schoolteacher and the child's school is essential for all hospitalised children. (**Good practice**)

continued

▶ Adolescent patients will require an additional profile of education plans, social issues and careers advice. The timing and practicalities of transition to adult units have to be actively discussed and planned. (**Good practice**)

Research and audit

Recommendation

▶ Each paediatric renal unit should maintain mortality and morbidity data for patients on HD. All vascular access related problems, such as catheter malfunction, exit site and tunnel infections, septicaemia rates, results of dialysis adequacy parameters and their relationship to growth, should be maintained by each unit. The data should be reported to the British Paediatric Renal Registry to be used for comparative audit and setting of standards. (**Good epidemiological practice**)

Access to and withdrawal from dialysis

Recommendation

▶ The decisions to institute active non-dialytic management of the patient in ESRD, including nutritional, medical and psychological support; or to discontinue dialysis already in train, should be made jointly by the patient and the responsible consultant nephrologist after consultation with relatives, the family practitioner and members of the caring team, abiding by the principles outlined briefly in chapter 3. The decision, and the reasons for it, must be recorded in the patient's notes. The numbers of patients not taken on to dialysis and the reasons for this decision should be subject to audit, as should the numbers and causes for those in whom dialysis is discontinued. Centres should develop guidelines for palliative care of such patients, including liaison with community services. (**Good practice**)

4 Peritoneal dialysis

Equipment and fluids*

Standards

▶ A unit offering peritoneal dialysis (PD) should provide not only continuous ambulatory peritoneal dialysis (CAPD) but also automated peritoneal dialysis (APD), in all its forms. It should have access to adequate back-up haemodialysis (HD) facilities and renal transplantation. (**Good practice**)

▶ All equipment used in the delivery and monitoring of therapies should comply with the relevant standards for medical electrical equipment (BS-EN 50072:1992, BS 5724-2.29:1992, IEC 60601-2-39:1998. Medical electrical equipment. Particular requirements for safety. Specification for peritoneal dialysis equipment). Tubing sets and catheters should carry the CE mark to indicate that the item conforms to the essential requirements of the Medical Devices Directive (93/42/EEC) and that its conformity has been assessed in accordance with the Directive. (**Good practice**)

*See Appendix D for details of standards abbreviations used in this chapter.

▶ Fluids for PD are required to satisfy the current European quality standards as indicated in the European good manufacturing practice and the European Pharmacopoeia Monograph, *Solutions for peritoneal dialysis*. Manufacturing facilities are required to meet the relevant standards (ISO 9001/2 and EN 46001/2). Product registration files must be submitted to, and product approval given by, the Medicines Control Agency. (**Good practice**)

▶ The use of disconnect systems should be standard unless clinically contraindicated. (**A**)

Recommendations

▶ The unit should be aware of the limitations of CAPD and related techniques. (**B**)

▶ In selected patients – (those with high small solute transfer rates and little or no residual function) – specialised solutions such as glucose polymers (icodextrin) are preferable to standard solutions. (**B**)

▶ Automated peritoneal dialysis (APD) should be available as clinically indicated and not constrained by financial considerations. (**C**)

Testing membrane function and dialysis adequacy

Recommendations

▶ A peritoneal equilibration test (PET) should be performed after 4–8 weeks on dialysis, and when clinically indicated, eg when biochemical indices or loss of ultrafiltration raise suspicion of changes in peritoneal transport characteristics, or when therapy is changed to APD. (**C**)

▶ A total weekly creatinine clearance (dialysis + residual renal function) of greater than 50 l/week/1.73 m^2 and/or a weekly dialysis Kt/V urea of greater than 1.7, checked eight weeks after beginning dialysis, are minima. Higher targets are desirable especially for high average and high transporters and APD patients. (**B**)

▶ At present both Kt/V and creatinine clearance are acceptable measures of adequacy until evidence accumulates to show the superiority of one over the other. Achieving either target is acceptable; creatinine clearance is more difficult to achieve in anuric patients with below average peritoneal solute transport. (**C**)

▶ These studies should be repeated at least annually, and more frequently if clinically indicated, particularly if suspicion arises that residual renal function has declined more rapidly than usual. (**C**)

▶ Careful attention to fluid balance, especially in anuric patients, is essential. The use of icodextrin in the day-time dwell combined with APD to achieve both adequate solute clearances and fluid removal is recommended. (**B**)

Infective complications

Recommendations

▶ Peritonitis rates should be <1 episode/18 patient months. (**A**)

▶ The negative peritoneal fluid culture rate in patients with clinical peritonitis should be less than 15%. (**B**)

▶ The initial cure rate of peritonitis should be more than 80% (without necessitating catheter removal). (**B**)

continued

▶ Mupirocin should be used as part of routine exit-site care; daily or on alternate days. **(B)**

▶ Nasal application of mupirocin in *Staphylococcus aureus* carriers should be undertaken twice daily for five consecutive days every four weeks. **(A)**

Paediatric section

Equipment, fluids and personnel

Standard

▶ All children requiring PD should be treated in a designated tertiary paediatric nephrology and dialysis centre. **(Good practice)**

Recommendations

▶ It is essential that the child and family are prepared for PD by a renally trained children's nurse with appropriate written information. Preparation by the nurse and/or play specialist will also include aids such as dolls or videos. **(Good practice)**

▶ Problems with needle phobia will require referral to a child psychologist. **(Good practice)**

▶ Insertion of the chronic peritoneal catheter should be by an appropriately trained surgeon. **(Good practice)**

▶ Training in the management of PD should be supervised by a paediatric renal nurse. **(Good practice)**

▶ The child's nutritional status needs to be managed and monitored by a paediatric renal dietitian. **(Good practice)**

▶ Since the home environment and the impact on the family are so important for the success of PD, psychosocial support such as liaison visits to the home, nursery or school and GP should be provided by the dialysis nurse and other team members such as social workers. **(Good practice)**

Testing membrane function and dialysis adequacy

Recommendations

▶ A PET and measurement of adequacy parameters should be undertaken annually but should be considered sooner if there is growth failure. **(Good practice)**

▶ Standards of adequacy recommended for adult patients should be regarded as the minimum for children. **(Good practice)**

Infective complications

Standard

▶ A minimum peritonitis rate of <1 episode per 14 patient months is recommended, averaged over three years. **(Good practice)**

Research and audit

> ### Recommendation
>
> ▶ Each paediatric renal unit should maintain mortality and morbidity data for patients on PD. All PD-related problems, such as catheter malfunction rates, exit site and tunnel infections and peritonitis rates, and results of dialysis adequacy parameters and their relationship to growth, should be maintained by each unit. The data should be submitted to the British Paediatric Renal Registry.

5 Haemodialysis and peritoneal dialysis: nutritional and biochemical standards

Albumin

> ### Recommendation
>
> ▶ Serum albumin should be measured regularly. A serum albumin concentration below 35 g/l, using a Bromocresol Green assay, or below 30 g/l using a Bromocresol Purple assay, should prompt clinical reassessment of the patient, looking for fluid overload, malnutrition, underdialysis, and remediable causes of an acute phase response. No audit standards can be set for measurements of serum albumin until there has been progress in standardisation of assays between different laboratories and in the understanding of the causes and appropriate treatment of hypoalbuminaemia in dialysis patients. (**Good practice**)

Bicarbonate

> ### Recommendations
>
> ▶ Serum bicarbonate, before a haemodialysis (HD) session, measured with minimal delay after venepuncture should be between 20 and 26 mmol/l. (**C**)
>
> ▶ For continuous ambulatory peritoneal dialysis (CAPD) patients serum bicarbonate, measured with minimal delay after venepuncture, should be between 25 and 29 mmol/l. (**B**)

Parathyroid hormone

> ### Standard
>
> ▶ Parathyroid hormone concentrations should be less than 4 times the upper limit of normal of the assay used in patients being managed for chronic renal failure or after transplantation and in patients who have been on HD or PD for longer than three months. (**B**)

Phosphate

> ### Standard
>
> ▶ Serum phosphate (measured before a dialysis session in HD patients) should be below 1.8 mmol/l. (**B**)

Calcium

▶ Serum calcium, adjusted for albumin concentration, should be between 2.2 and 2.6 mmol/l, in HD (pre-dialysis sample) patients and in PD patients. **(B)**

Potassium

Standard

▶ Pre-dialysis serum potassium should be between 3.5 and 6.5 mmol/l in HD patients. Serum potassium should be between 3.5 and 5.5 mmol/l in PD patients. **(Good practice)**

Aluminium

Recommendation

▶ Serum aluminium concentration should be measured every three months in all patients on HD and in all PD patients receiving oral aluminium hydroxide. No patient whose ferritin level is <100 μg/l should have a serum aluminium concentration >60 μg/l (2.2 μmol/l). **(B)**

Nutritional screening

Standard

▶ All patients with ESRD both before and after the start of dialysis should undergo regular screening for undernutrition. **(Good practice)**

Recommendations

▶ Nutritional screening should include as a minimum subjective global assessment (SGA) measurement of height, weight and serum albumin. Body mass index (BMI) should be calculated (weight in kilograms divided by the square of the height in metres) and unintentional loss of oedema free weight recorded. **(Good practice)**

▶ A diagnosis of undernutrition should be considered if any one of the following criteria are met:
  – BMI < 18.5
  – unintentional loss of oedema free weight >10% in past six months
  – albumin < 35 g/l (bromocresol green) or < 30 g/l (bromocresol purple) **(B)**
  – SGA scores of 1–2 (severe undernutrition) or 3–5 (mild to moderate undernutrition). **(Good practice)**

Assessment of nutritional status in undernourished patients

Recommendation

▶ If a diagnosis of undernutrition is suspected on the above criteria then a full nutritional assessment should be undertaken by a clinician and renal dietitian to elucidate the underlying cause. This should include a full medical history, assessment of dietary intake (three-day dietary record and measurement of the protein equivalent of nitrogen appearance), measurement of CRP, serum bicarbonate and measurement of dialysis adequacy and residual renal function. **(Good practice)**

Management of malnutrition

Recommendations

▶ In all patients found to have an inadequate dietary intake, identifiable causes should be corrected and dietary advice given to increase intake. Oral supplements, intraperitoneal amino acids (IPAA – CAPD), intradialytic parenteral nutrition (IDPN – HD), nasogastric (NG) feeding, percutaneous endoscopic gastrostomy (PEG) feeding and intravenous partial/total parenteral nutrition are all recognised means by which dietary intake can be supplemented. Local protocols incorporating these methods should be agreed. **(Good practice)**

▶ In those patients found to have a persistently high CRP, a source of infection should be sought and treated. **(Good practice)**

▶ Where dietary intake is adequate, catabolic factors such as acidosis, thyrotoxicosis and uncontrolled diabetes should be sought and treated. **(Good practice)**

Dietary sodium intake

Recommendation

▶ All patients with ESRD both before and after the start of dialysis should be advised to limit dietary salt intake to less than 6 g/day (equivalent to approximately 100 mmol of sodium). **(B)**

Obesity

Recommendation

▶ All patients with chronic renal failure should receive dietary advice to avoid weight gain beyond a BMI >30. **(C)**

Paediatric section

Parathyroid hormone (PTH), phosphate and calcium

Standard

▶ Serum phosphate and calcium should be kept within the normal range. PTH levels should be maintained within twice the upper limit of the normal range but, contrary to adult standards, may be kept within the normal range if growth is normal. **(B)**

Nutritional management and growth

Standards

▶ Measures of supine length or standing height and weight should be monitored at each clinic visit. Head circumference should be measured at each visit before 2 years of age and six monthly up to 5 years of age. All measurements should be plotted on reference European growth charts for healthy children. The data should be returned to the UK Renal Registry every six months. **(Good practice)**

▶ All children should undergo dietary assessment by a paediatric renal dietitian at a minimum of every three months, but more often if there is deteriorating biochemistry or growth. Inadequate intake should be supplemented orally or enterally. **(Good practice)**

continued

▶ Recombinant human growth hormone (rhGH) may be offered to children of all ages who have a height standard deviation score (Ht SDS) more than 2 SD below the mean (or below the 2nd percentile), and a height velocity SDS less than the 25th centile, whose growth has failed to respond to adequate nutrition, correction of metabolic abnormalities, adequate dialysis and, if post transplant, reduction of prednisolone to a minimum. **(B)**

Sodium intake

Recommendation

▶ Many children with CRF have renal dysplasia with renal tubular losses of salt and water that may require salt supplementation. **(C)**

6 Cardiovascular risk factors in patients on dialysis

Blood pressure

Standards

▶ Pre-haemodialysis systolic blood pressure should be below 140 mmHg. **(C)**

▶ Pre-haemodialysis diastolic blood pressure should be below 90 mmHg. **(C)**

▶ Post-dialysis systolic blood pressure should be below 130 mmHg. **(C)**

▶ Post-dialysis diastolic blood pressure should be below 80 mmHg. **(C)**

▶ Post-dialysis blood pressure should be recorded after completion of dialysis, including washback. **(Good practice)**

▶ Blood pressure in patients on peritoneal dialysis should be below 130 mmHg systolic and 80 mmHg diastolic. **(C)**

Recommendation

▶ Blood pressure should be measured according to the recommendations of the British Hypertension Society, in the non-fistula arm with an appropriate cuff size, with the patient seated comfortably for five minutes prior to measurement; following 30 minutes abstention from caffeine and nicotine. The arm should be supported at heart level and at least two measurements of blood pressure are taken, either with a mercury sphygmomanometer or with a validated electronic device. A third should be taken if there is a significant discrepancy between the first two. The mean of the last two measurements should be recorded. **(Good practice)**

Identification and management of cardiac dysfunction

Recommendation

▶ All dialysis patients should have unimpeded access to echocardiography for the identification of LVH and LV dysfunction. **(Good practice)**

Identification and treatment of left ventricular failure

Recommendations

▶ All dialysis units should record the development of left ventricular failure (see explanation in chapter 6.15) in a manner permitting audit of the management of such patients. (**Good practice**)

▶ All patients with suspected heart failure should be investigated using echocardiography. (**Good practice**)

▶ All patients with proven systolic heart failure should receive treatment with angiotensin converting enzyme (ACE) inhibitors and low-dose beta-blockers unless specifically contraindicated. (**B**)

Primary prevention of atherosclerotic cardiovascular disease

Recommendations

▶ Smoking habit should be recorded in dialysis patients in a manner permitting audit and should be actively discouraged in all those with a reasonable life expectancy and strongly discouraged in those on the transplant waiting list. (**Good practice**)

▶ Exercise should be encouraged. (**Good practice**)

▶ Glycosated haemoglobin (HbA1c) should be below 7% in dialysis patients with diabetes, measured using an assay method which has been harmonised to the Diabetes Control and Complication Trial (DCCT) standard. (**B**)

▶ 3-hydroxy-3 methylglutary–Co-enzyme A (HMG–CoA) reductase inhibitors should be considered for primary prevention in dialysis patients with a 10-year risk of coronary disease, calculated according to the Joint British Societies Chart or the Coronary Risk Calculator, of ≥30%, ignoring the fact that these calculations may not be accurate in patients with renal disease. A total cholesterol of <5 mmol/l or a 30% reduction from baseline, or a fasting LDL-cholesterol of < 3 mmol/l should be achieved, whichever is the greater reduction. (**C**)

▶ HMG-CoA reductase inhibitors should not be withdrawn from patients in whom they were previously indicated and prescribed when such patients start renal replacement therapy (RRT) or change modality. (**C**)

▶ Serum or red cell folate should be above the lower limit of the reference range in patients on dialysis. (**Good practice**)

Secondary prevention of ischaemic heart disease

Recommendations

▶ All dialysis units should record myocardial infarction, stroke, transient ischaemic attacks, and symptomatic peripheral vascular disease events in a manner permitting audit of the management of such patients. (**Good practice**)

▶ All dialysis patients with a history of myocardial infarction, stroke, peripheral vascular disease, acute coronary syndrome, or who undergo surgical or angiographic coronary revascularisation should be treated with aspirin, an ACE inhibitor, a beta-blocker, and an HMG–CoA reductase inhibitor unless contraindicated. Doses of ACE inhibitors and beta-blockers should be the maximum tolerated. (**C**)

▶ In patients in whom lipid-lowering drug treatment is used, total cholesterol should be reduced by 30% or to below 5 mmol/l, or LDL-cholesterol to below 3 mmol/l whichever reduction is the greatest. (**C**)

continued

▶ Dialysis patients should have unimpeded access to a full range of cardiac investigations including exercise echocardiography, radio-isotopic cardiac scans, and coronary angiography. (**Good practice**)

Paediatric section

Blood pressure

Standard

▶ Blood pressure varies throughout childhood and should be maintained within two standard deviations of the mean for normal children of the same height and sex. (**C**)

Recommendations

▶ The systolic blood pressure during pre-terminal CRF should be maintained at <90th centile for age, gender and height. (**C**)

▶ The systolic blood pressure during PD should be maintained at <90th centile for age, gender and height. Parents should be taught blood pressure recording and provided with appropriate equipment for measurement at home. (**C**)

▶ The systolic blood pressure after HD should be maintained at <90th centile for age, gender and height. In those with sustained hypertension, parents should be taught blood pressure recording and provided with appropriate equipment for measurement on the days between dialyses as this may be more representative of overall control than pre-dialysis blood pressure. (**C**)

▶ 'Whitecoat' hypertension does occur in children and is compounded by the pressure effect of the automated blood pressure devices. Twenty-four hour ambulatory blood pressure monitoring in children should be available in all tertiary paediatric centres. (**Good practice**)

▶ Echocardiography in hypertensive patients is recommended at yearly intervals as a minimum. (**Good practice**)

Lipids

Recommendations

▶ Fasting cholesterol and trigylceride levels should be measured in all children commencing renal replacement therapy and at annual intervals. (**Good practice**)

▶ The dietetic advice from the paediatric renal dietitian for children over two years of age should take into consideration nutritional guidelines on cardiovascular disease and the document *The balance of good health*. (**C**)

7 Anaemia in patients with chronic renal failure

Standards

▶ Target haemoglobin. Patients with chronic renal failure (CRF) should achieve a haemoglobin of 10 g/dl **(A)*** within six months of being seen by a nephrologist, unless there is a specific reason such as those outlined below. It is unclear as yet how epoetin should be used optimally in patients before dialysis becomes necessary and whether normalisation of haemoglobin gives further benefit.

▶ Adequate iron status. Patients must be iron replete to achieve and maintain target haemoglobin whether receiving epoetin or not. **(B)** A definition of adequate iron status is a serum ferritin >100 µg/l and <10% hypochromic red cells (transferrin saturation >20%)**.

Recommendations

▶ Evaluate anaemia in CRF when Hb<12 g/dl (adult males and post- menopausal females), <11 g/dl (pre-menopausal females) **(B)**; anaemia may be considered the result of uraemia if the GFR is <30 ml/min (<45/ml/min in diabetics) and no other cause, eg blood loss, folate or B12 deficiency, is identified. **(B)**

▶ Iron administration: oral iron will in general be sufficient to attain and maintain the above targets in those not yet requiring dialysis and those on peritoneal dialysis (PD); in contrast, many haemodialysis (HD) patients will require intravenous iron. **(B)**

▶ Regular monitoring of iron status (at least every six months) is essential during treatment to avoid toxicity: a serum ferritin consistently greater than 800 µg/l is suggestive of iron overload. **(B)**

▶ Route of epoetin administration: it is preferable to give epoetin subcutaneously even in HD patients. **(A)** Some patients (such as obese subjects) may require intravenous injection to obtain good absorption.

▶ Haemoglobin concentration should be monitored monthly for stable hospital haemodialysis patients and 3 to 4 monthly for stable home HD and PD patients and epoetin dosage adjusted accordingly. **(C)** Haemoglobin will require to be monitored more frequently to begin with.

▶ 'Resistance' to epoetin: failure to reach the target, or need for doses of epoetin above 300 IU/kg/week, defines inadequate response ('resistance'). Iron deficiency (absolute or functional) remains the commonest cause. Hyporesponsive patients who are iron replete should be screened clinically and by laboratory testing for other common causes, such as raised iPTH, malignancy, infection/inflammation, aluminium toxicity, effect of ACE inhibitors and possibly epoetin antibodies. **(B)**

▶ Blood pressure: must be monitored in all patients receiving epoetin and hypertension if present (for definition see Chapter 6) should be treated by volume removal and/or hypotensive drugs. **(B)**

---

* Level A evidence so far only for dialysis patients.
** Pre-dialysis blood sample in those on haemodialysis.

Paediatric section

Standards

▶ Target haemoglobin: all children with CRF and on dialysis should achieve their target haemoglobin within six months of seeing a paediatric nephrologist, unless there is a specific reason otherwise. Targets are age specific, as below:

- ▶ Children under six months of age should achieve a haemoglobin of greater than or equal to 9.5 g/dl.

- ▶ Children aged six months to two years should achieve a haemoglobin of greater than or equal to 10.0 g/dl.

- ▶ Children over two years of age should achieve a haemoglobin of greater than or equal to 10.5 g/dl. **(B)**

▶ Adequate iron status: all children should achieve a serum ferritin of greater than 100 μg/l and less than 800 μg/l, whether or not they are receiving epoetin. **(B)**

Recommendations

▶ Evaluation of anaemia: the haemoglobin rises throughout childhood as follows: normal range (±2 SD) before six months of age is 11.5 (9.5–13.5) g/dl; from six months to two years it is 12.0 (10.5–13.5) g/dl; and it rises progressively to 13.5 (11.5–15.5) g/dl by 12 years. Evaluate for anaemia when the haemoglobin falls to <10 g/dl before six months of age, <11 g/dl from six months to two years, and <12 g/dl in older children. **(Good practice)**

▶ Iron administration: persistently low ferritin despite oral supplementation is an indication for intravenous iron therapy. Side effects must be monitored. **(B)**

▶ Haemoglobin concentration should be monitored every 1–2 months. **(Good practice)**

▶ Iron status should be monitored every three months. **(Good practice)**

8 Transplantation

Access to transplantation and allocation of kidneys

Standards

▶ There must be demonstrable equity of access to donor organs irrespective of gender, race or district of residence. Age in itself is not a contraindication to transplantation but age-related morbidity is important. **(Good practice)**

▶ All transplant units should have written criteria for acceptance on to the waiting list for renal transplantation and all patients on dialysis should be offered the opportunity of assessment by nephrologists, transplant surgeons and transplant coordinators who should explain whether or not they are suitable for transplantation. The risks associated with transplantation should be fully explained verbally and in writing. **(Good practice)**

▶ All dialysis patients should have their suitability for transplantation reviewed at least annually and recorded. Patients should be placed on or removed from transplant waiting lists only after discussion and agreement with nephrologists, transplant surgeons and the patients themselves. (**Good practice**)

▶ Kidneys should be allocated according to nationally agreed guidelines that take account of matching, waiting time, sensitisation and other factors. (**Good practice**)

Organ donation rate/living donor transplantation

Recommendations

▶ Services for kidney retrieval must be an integral part of organ transplant services and costed into them. (**Good practice**)

▶ Purchasers should fund efforts to increase the number of cadaver organs made available by the setting up of transplant co-ordination and organ procurement teams and they should ensure that adequate educational programmes are in place; an important part of this is improved communication with intensive care units. (**Good practice**)

▶ An increase in live donor transplantation should be actively encouraged and living donors should remain under life-long follow-up. (**Good practice**)

The transplant unit

Recommendations

▶ Transplant units should in general serve at least two million total population, depending on geography, communications and population density. They should be appropriately located and preferably perform at least 50 transplants per year. (**Good practice**)

▶ Transplant Units must be adequately staffed both medically and surgically at senior and junior level, and have full support services including a pathologist trained in the interpretation of renal transplant biopsies. Specialist advisory committee recommendations and junior doctors' hours guidelines must be followed. (**Good practice**)

▶ The care of the renal transplant recipient is best carried out by a multidisciplinary team with equal input from nephrologists and transplant surgeons. This element of care along with full integration with the dialysis service, is essential. (**Good practice**)

Blood pressure

Standard

▶ Blood pressure targets for renal transplant recipients are <130 mmHg systolic and <80 mmHg diastolic. (**B**)

Histocompatibility matching and allocation of donor kidneys

Standards

▶ Sensitised recipients must have the HLA-specificities of circulating antibodies defined carefully. The sensitisation status of every patient registered on the national waiting list should be reviewed on at least an annual basis. (**B**)

▶ All donor recipient pairs should be cross-matched by an appropriate technique before transplantation. Flow cytometric cross-matching may be helpful for re-transplants and highly sensitised recipients. (**B**)

▶ An accredited tissue typing service is an essential part of a successful kidney transplant programme. Day-to-day direction of the laboratory must be provided by a medical or scientific consultant trained in histocompatibility and immunogenetics (H&I). The tissue typing laboratory staff must be an integral part of the transplant team. Laboratory staff must be available 24 hours a day to type and cross-match against donors. Living donors and recipients must be tested as required under the terms of the Human Organ Transplants Act 1989. (**Good practice**)

▶ All centres should document local allocation criteria. Patient registration on the national waiting list must contain sufficient HLA typing and sensitisation information to support the operation of the allocation scheme. (**Good practice**)

▶ All screening for HLA-specific antibodies should use a typed panel that allows interpretation of positive reactions. The tissue-typing laboratory must be provided with patients' serum following sensitising events such as the transfusion of blood products or transplantation. Following transplantation it is essential that the tissue-typing laboratory continues regularly to receive serum samples for antibody screening. Failure to provide these samples may jeopardise a patient's future chances of transplantation. All potential recipients must be screened regularly for HLA-specific antibodies. This should be at least every three months. (**Good practice**)

Immuno-suppressive regimens and early complications

Standard

▶ Transplant units should provide written documentation on agreed policies regarding immunosuppressive protocols, prophylaxis against cytomegalovirus, pneumocystis and renal vein thrombosis and management of delayed graft function. Such protocols should be reviewed annually in the light of published research and in-house experience. (**Good practice**)

Clinical outcome and audit

Standards

▶ Organs should be retrieved from at least 15 heart beating donors per million population per year. Each unit should transplant at least 25 patients per million population per year using cadaver kidneys. Efforts should be made to limit the cold ischaemic time to less than 30 hours in all cases and to much less than 24 hours wherever possible. Each transplant unit which has appropriate resources to perform live donor transplantation should transplant a minimum of five living donor grafts per million population per year, but it is hoped that a higher number than this can be achieved in the future. At least 60% of recipients of cadaveric grafts should receive a 000 mismatch or other favourable matched kidney. (**Good practice**)

▶ At least 70% of heart beating cadaver kidney transplants should function immediately, and at least 95% should function eventually. Graft survival of second grafts should be the same as for first grafts, provided that adequate analysis of alloantibodies and fluorescence activated cell sorter (FACS) cross-matching are used. There should be at least 95% patient survival at 1 year after transplantation for recipients of live donor and cadaveric kidneys. More than 84% of cadaver grafts and 90% of live grafts should still be working at 1 year and at least 68% of cadaver grafts and 73% of live donor grafts should still be working at five years. (**Good practice**)

Paediatric section

Access to transplantation and allocation of kidneys

Standards

▶ All children under 15 years of age being prepared for or undergoing transplantation should be cared for in a paediatric nephrology centre. **(Good practice)**

▶ The UKT scheme giving priority to children for favourably matched kidneys should continue. **(Good practice)**

Recommendations

▶ Pre-emptive transplantation should be encouraged as it conserves peritoneal and vascular access for future use and improves growth. **(Good practice)**

▶ Living related donor transplantation should be encouraged. **(Good practice)**

Organ donation/ living donor transplantation

Recommendation

▶ The use of kidneys from donors under the age of five years or over 55 years is not recommended in paediatric patients. **(B)**

The transplant unit

Recommendation

▶ There should be 24-hour access to a consultant paediatric nephrologist, transplant surgeon, urologist, general surgeon, anaesthetist and intensivist. **(Good practice)**

Histocompatibility matching and allocation of donor kidneys

Recommendation

▶ Centres should aim for at least 60% of kidneys being favourably matched. **(B)**

Immuno-suppressive regimens and early complications

Recommendation

▶ Centres should be encouraged to enter patients into prospective randomised paediatric trials to assess the efficacy, safety and tolerability of new immunosuppressive agents. **(Good practice)**

Transfer of patients to adult service

Recommendation

▶ All centres should have a written policy for the transfer of adolescents to adult units. **(Good practice)**

Clinical outcome and audit

▶ Each unit should report their data to the Paediatric Renal Registry to enable annual national assessment of outcomes of paediatric transplantation. (**Good epidemiological practice**)

▶ Centres should audit each graft loss to identify possible avoidable factors. (**Good practice**)

9 Blood-borne viruses and microbiology in the renal unit

Good working practices

Recommendation

▶ The general and universal precautions described below should be observed. (**Good practice**)

Immunisation and patient testing

Recommendations

▶ Patients awaiting start of ESRD treatment should be immunised against HBV as soon as possible while their plasma creatinine remains relatively low. (**B**)

▶ All long-term dialysis patients should be immunised against HBV. Those who develop an adequate antibody response should be given a booster dose of vaccine every five years. As there is evidence that poor responders derive some benefit from vaccination, they should be given a booster after one year and every five years thereafter. Non-responders should receive a repeat course of vaccine. (**B**)

▶ Testing should be carried out three monthly for HBsAg, and HCV antibody and annually for HIV antibody. An annual test for HBs Ag is sufficient for patients who have demonstrated immunity. More frequent testing is appropriate in those exposed to blood-borne viruses (BBVs). (**Good practice**)

▶ Hepatitis B immunoglobulin and vaccine should be given, if appropriate, to susceptible patients who have been exposed to the virus. (**B**)

▶ The patient's informed consent to testing should be obtained. Those who withhold consent or who are incapable of giving consent should be managed as though they were BBV infected. However, infected patients should not be denied dialysis. (**Good practice**)

Management of patients carrying BBVs

Recommendations

▶ Whenever possible, staff should care for only BBV-infected or uninfected patients during one shift. If this is not practicable, the more experienced staff should be assigned the task of caring for a mixed group of patients. Designated staff should nurse affected patients when there has been an outbreak of BBV infection in a unit. In the case of hepatitis B, staff who demonstrated immunity should care for the patients whenever possible. (**Good practice**)

▶ Carriers of hepatitis B should be dialysed in separate rooms on dedicated machines. (**Good practice**)

► Carriers of hepatitis C should be dialysed in separate shifts and units should move towards providing separate rooms for such patients. **(Good practice)**

► Dialysis machines used for patients positive for hepatitis C may be used for other patients provided that the dialysis circuit has been adequately decontaminated and the external surface cleaned with some suitable disinfectant between patient use. **(Good practice)**

► Segregation of HIV-infected patients should be considered, based on local risk assessment. Their machines should be treated as for patients with Hepatitis C. **(Good practice)**

Dialysis personnel and BBVs

Standards

► Staff working in dialysis units in contact with patients, machines or materials used in dialysis should show immunity to HBV. Non-, or poor responders should be tested annually for HBs antigen and antibody to HB core antigen. Staff who are positive for HBsAg should demonstrate they are not HBe antigen positive or are HBe antigen negative with a viral load of less than 10^3 genome equivalents per ml. Non-clinical staff need not be tested for BBVs. **(Good practice)**

► There is no need to screen for HCV or HIV in staff, but those known to be at risk of acquiring infection or known to be infected should be encouraged to seek advice from an occupational health physician. **(Good practice)**

Staphylococcus aureus (SA) infection control in dialysis units

Recommendations

► All units should have a documented infection control policy covering general measures together with specific advice on limiting SA-related infections and preventing the spread of MRSA and other multi-resistant strains. This will usually be developed in conjunction with the hospital infection control unit. Key features should include guidelines for screening to detect nasal carriage, prophylactic therapy in different dialysis populations, antibiotic therapy for presumed *staphylococcal* infections, staff and patient education, an emphasis on the importance of hand washing and an isolation policy for MRSA carriers admitted to hospital. **(Good practice)**

► All dialysis patients should be screened on a three-monthly basis for SA nasal carriage. **(Good practice)**

► Patients undergoing haemodialysis via a temporary central venous dialysis catheter should have either 2% mupirocin ointment **(A)** or povidone-iodine ointment **(A)** applied to the cannula exit site after insertion and at the end of each dialysis session.

► All HD patients who are SA nasal carriers should receive either eradication therapy with a course of intranasal 2% mupirocin cream **(Good practice)** or eradication therapy followed by long-term once-weekly application of 2% mupirocin cream. **(A)**

► Patients on peritoneal dialysis should apply 2% mupirocin ointment to the exit site on a daily or alternate daily basis as part of routine exit-site care. **(B)**

► Patients on PD who are SA nasal carriers should receive either eradication therapy with a course of intranasal 2% mupirocin cream **(Good practice)** or have regular five-day courses of intranasal 2% mupirocin every four weeks. **(A)**

10 The management of patients approaching end-stage renal disease (ESRD)

Recommendation

▶ Patients with progressive renal failure should be managed in a clinic with multidisciplinary support from dieticians and specialist nurses. (**Good practice**)

Blood pressure control

Standards

▶ Blood pressure targets are 125/75 mmHg for those with progressive proteinuric renal disease and 130/80 mmHg for those with stable renal function. (**A**)

▶ Angiotensin converting enzyme (ACE) inhibitors should be considered as the agents of first choice in the management of hypertension in patients with progressive renal disease. (**A**)

Recommendations

▶ Patients should be advised where necessary to stop smoking. (**B**)

▶ Patients should be advised where necessary to reduce dietary salt intake, take regular exercise, and reduce alcohol intake. (**C**)

Nutritional management

Recommendations

▶ Patients should be advised where necessary to lose weight, reduce dietary salt intake, and take regular exercise. (**Good practice**)

▶ Dietary protein intake should be approximately 0.75 g/kg/day. (**B**)

▶ Patients should be regularly screened for undernutrition. (**Good practice**)

▶ Serum bicarbonate should be in the normal range. (**C**)

▶ Serum phosphate should be <1.9 mmol/l. (**B**)

Initiation of dialysis

Recommendations

▶ Dialysis should be considered when the weekly urea clearance falls below the equivalent of a *Kt/V* of 2.0 (equivalent to a GFR of approximately 14 ml/min). Dialysis will be indicated in such patients if there is evidence of malnutrition or if symptoms interfere which quality of life. It is prudent to consider dialysis at this early stage in those with predictably steadily progressive renal failure as occurs in polycystic disease or glomerulonephritis. Those with relatively stable renal function, however, may often be treated conservatively. (**Good practice**)

▶ All patients should be able to start dialysis when clinically indicated; there should be no waiting list for dialysis. (**Good practice**)

▶ Patients with progressive renal failure should be referred to a nephrologist early in the course of their disease (serum creatinine 150–200 μmol/l) to enable dialysis to be started in a planned fashion. (**Good practice**)

Paediatric section

Indications for initiation of dialysis

Standards

▶ All children should be offered dialysis if their measured or calculated GFR falls to 10–15 ml/min/1.73m^2 unless the child remains asymptomatic and growth is well maintained. (**Good practice**)

▶ Pre-emptive transplantation should be offered to children in whom the progressive decline in renal function gives sufficient time to prepare them for the transplant list, as transplantation is the goal for all children with ESRD. (**Good practice**)

Recommendation

▶ Paediatric renal units should supply data to the Paediatric Renal Registry, including the time of referral to the paediatric renal unit with growth parameters at that time. Similar indices should be recorded at the time of initiation of dialysis or pre-emptive transplantation. This will provide data for informed discussion about ways of improving late referral and timing of renal replacement therapy (RRT) intervention. (**Good epidemiological practice**)

Standards

▶ All children should complete a standard course of childhood immunisation as stipulated by the Department of Health. (**C**)

▶ Each unit should have an immunisation policy. It is recommended that hepatitis B, varicella and BCG vaccination after Heaf testing are completed prior to transplantation. (**Good practice**)

Nursing and family support

Standards

▶ All children should be cared for by paediatric nephrology nurses, who deliver specialised care for children who need RRT both in hospital and in the community. (**Good practice**)

▶ Prior to commencing home peritoneal dialysis, a home assessment should be undertaken. (**Good practice**)

▶ All families should have access to other staff who may be involved in the care of the child with chronic renal failure, including play staff, schoolteachers, psychologists, psychiatrists and youth workers. (**Good practice**)

▶ All children and families should have access to support from members of the multidisciplinary team. Their information needs should be assessed and met via interviews, booklets, videos and other resources. It is important that phobias, particularly needle phobias, are addressed as these can assume immense importance in the long-term care of a child on RRT. (**Good practice**)

11 Acute renal failure

Where patients should be managed?

Recommendations

▶ Renal wards admitting patients with acute renal failure (ARF) require either a designated High Dependency Unit (HDU) or access to a centralised HDU where, in addition to renal replacement therapy (RRT), the following are available: close nursing supervision, oxygen, continuous electrocardiogram (ECG) and oxygen saturation monitoring, automated blood pressure (BP) monitoring, and central venous pressure (CVP) monitoring facilities and expertise. There should be provision for dialysis on alternate days for all patients with ARF and for daily dialysis for those who require it. (**Good practice**)

▶ Patients with multiple organ failure and those who are haemodynamically very unstable should be managed on an intensive care unit (ICU), and be transferred there in a timely manner. (**Good practice**)

▶ Whilst it is reasonable for patients with uncomplicated ARF to receive dialysis on a chronic dialysis unit, it is bad practice for this to be done without adequate on-site medical supervision. (**Good practice**)

Techniques of treatment and when to start

Recommendation

▶ Treatment of haemodynamically unstable patients with ARF requires continuous treatment techniques and the facilities of an ICU. (**Good practice**)

Access to specialist nephrological services

Recommendations

▶ In hospitals with both a renal unit and an ICU, patients with multiple organ failure including ARF should be managed jointly by intensive care physicians and nephrologists. (**Good practice**)

▶ All those supervising RRT should have received adequate training. (**Good practice**)

▶ All ICUs without in-house access to a renal unit should have formal links with a named renal unit for advice and consultation, which should be sought for all appropriate patients. This commitment has workload and staffing implications for renal units. (**Good practice**)

Paediatric section

▶ All children with ARF require discussion with a paediatric nephrologist. Early transfer for investigation and management is essential in those with rapidly deteriorating renal function or in those with haemodynamic or biochemical disturbances. Children with ARF and multi-organ failure require transfer to a designated regional paediatric ICU lead centre. Although most children with ARF recover renal function, nephrological follow-up during childhood is often necessary as the long-term prognosis is uncertain. (**Good practice**)

▶ Where children with ARF are provided with dialysis by adult nephrologists for reasons of geography, the child should be primarily under the care of a paediatrician, who will consult when necessary with the regional paediatric unit and discuss complications at an early stage. Transfer to a regional unit is indicated if there is progression to multi-system disease or if it is evident that the child is has reached end-stage renal failure. (**Good practice**)

1 | Methods of guideline development

The process of producing the standards document

1.1   The second edition of this document was reviewed by the Health Care Evaluation Unit of the Department of Public Health Sciences at St George's Hospital Medical School using their *Appraisal instrument for clinical guidelines*.[1] Their suggestions were, as far as possible, incorporated into this document, and their schema was used to develop this edition.

Responsibility for guideline development

1.2   In November 1997 the Renal Association in conjunction with the Royal College of Physicians of London convened the Standards and Audit Subcommittee to produce the third edition of *Treatment of adult patients with renal failure – recommended standards and audit measures*. The Renal Association provided funding for travel to meetings and for a small exploratory literature search. Members of the Subcommittee wrote the chapters in their own time. It was decided to cover the care of children more fully in this document and hence there is a paediatric section to complement each chapter. Consequently the title of the document has been changed to *Treatment of adults and children with renal failure – standards and audit measures*. The chapter on transplantation was written jointly by the Standards and Audit Subcommittee and the British Transplantation Society. The chapter on acute renal failure was written in conjunction with the Intensive Care Society, a member of which was on the Standards and Audit Subcommittee. All paediatric sections were written along with members of the British Association of Paediatric Nephrology (BAPN) which also had representation on the Subcommittee.

Guideline development group

1.3   The membership of the Subcommittee was expanded for this edition of the document (for a full membership list see page iii). There was representation from the National Federation of Kidney Patients Associations, nursing staff, medical staff caring for adults and children with renal disease, public health medicine, the UK Renal Registry, NHS management, the Royal College of Physicians of London and the Renal Association. Members of the Departments of Health of England, Wales, Northern Ireland and Scotland were present as observers.

Identification and interpretation of the evidence

1.4   The standards and recommendations in this document vary in their underlying nature and hence in the types of evidence required. There are six main types:

a)   **The optimal interventions to use** (eg which membrane for haemodialysis).

b)   **Target values of intermediate patient outcomes** (eg haemoglobin, phosphate, bicarbonate).

c)   **Epidemiological data** (eg about population need).

d)   **Statistical methodology** (eg outcomes data).

e)   **Organisation of services** (eg how many transplant units for a given population base).

f) **Good clinical practice, particularly with regard to ethical issues** (eg the decision to withhold or withdraw dialysis should be made after consultation with the patient and his/her family).

These are described in greater detail below.

a) The optimal interventions to use

For most interventions the best type of evidence is the randomised controlled trial. If several trials have addressed one question they can be subject to systematic review that may or may not incorporate a meta-analysis. These are available on the Cochrane database of reviews (www.cochrane.co.uk) or the York Centre for Reviews & Dissemination (CRD) Database of Abstracts of Reviews of Effectiveness (DARE) database (www.york.ac.uk/inst/crd). Compared with many areas of medicine, particularly cardiology, stroke medicine and oncology, there are relatively few trials in patients with renal failure which record patient-centred outcomes (including survival, quality of life and hospitalisation rates) and have sufficiently long follow-up. The paucity of such trials may in part reflect the smaller number of patients with renal failure, particularly end stage renal disease (ESRD), but there is a need routinely to test new drugs and technologies for such patients in trials as is done for those, for example, with haematological malignancy. This may be particularly difficult, however, for interventions in the small number of children with ESRD.

The above databases were searched for relevant topics for all chapters and subsequent papers retrieved and forwarded to the writers of the chapters for appraisal and inclusion where appropriate. We aimed also to review the evidence from relevant trials using databases such as Medline or Embase but we had insufficient resources. However, a formal search for publications on the treatment of hypertension was made. Our evidence-based approach was supported by the National Institute of Clinical Excellence (NICE) although they had no funding available at that time. A grant application was therefore submitted to the National Kidney Research Fund to review the evidence base for questions selected by the Standards and Audit Subcommittee. This grant was subsequently awarded and the systematic reviews produced will provide an improved evidence base for future editions of this document.

The chapter authors therefore searched the literature, often using Medline in the manner of the previous edition. Trials and retrospective and prospective cohort studies were the principle sources and the evidence was graded using the system of the US Department of Health and Human Services (Table 1).[2]

b) Target values of intermediate patient outcomes

Several of the standards are values of intermediate patient outcomes (eg haemoglobin, serum phosphate). Randomised trials can be carried out for such values, particularly where one or two major interventions can markedly influence the value, eg the influence of epoetin and iron therapies on haemoglobin values. Patients can be randomised to two target haemoglobin ranges and outcomes compared. In contrast, serum potassium values must be kept within a narrow range to maintain life and hence a trial would be entirely inappropriate.

Other indices, eg serum phosphate and serum bicarbonate values, may be useful indicators of the quality of the overall process of dialysis care reflecting the effect of diet, drug therapy and/or length and nature of dialysis treatment. Trials of target ranges would be theoretically possible, but since they reflect many aspects of treatment, altering phosphate levels in isolation may not improve the outcome for the patient. Achieved values may vary between countries, and in part reflect the resources invested in dialysis therapy, hence cohort studies require cautious interpretation.

Trials and cohort studies where available, were evaluated by chapter authors. Evidence levels quoted in Table 1 are used where appropriate. Other recommendations are termed 'good practice'.

Table 1. Strength of recommendations:

A = Evidence from at least one properly performed randomised controlled trial (**quality of evidence Ib**) or meta-analysis of several controlled trials (**quality of evidence Ia**).

B = Well conducted clinical studies, but no randomised clinical trials; evidence may be extensive but essentially descriptive (**evidence levels IIa, IIb, III**).

C = Evidence (**level IV**) obtained from expert committee reports or opinions, and/or clinical experience of respected authorities. This grading indicates an absence of directly applicable studies of good quality.

c/d) Epidemiological data (eg about population need) and statistical methodology (eg outcomes data)

Important standards concern the population needs for treatment and the ways in which data on patients with renal failure should be monitored and statistically analysed, eg data on patients with end stage renal disease should be recorded by the UK Renal Registry. Such standards have been defined for this edition as 'good statistical practice' or 'good epidemiological practice'.

e) Organisation of services (eg how many transplant units for a given population base)

Several standards concern the organisation and delivery of services for patients with renal failure. Optimally the evidence-based clinical standards should serve as building blocks for standards of service provision. For example, a clinical standard indicating a target value for haemoglobin could translate into a service provision standard of adequate epoetin and iron provision and appropriate staffing to deliver that standard. The evidence base for many aspects of care of patients with renal failure still requires to be determined and hence the standards of service provision quoted are frequently based on consensus. For other service standards a consensus view is the appropriate and only sensible way to establish them. This consensus was obtained, following discussion, at the meetings of the multidisciplinary Standards and Audit Subcommittee.

f) Good clinical practice, and particularly with regard to ethical issues

Some standards concern ethical issues and these recommendations are termed 'good practice' as described in section (b) above.

Formulation of recommendations

1.5   The document was divided into chapters and one, or more frequently two, members of the group who had a particular experience or interest in the area were selected to write each chapter. They in turn could (if they wished) invite other colleagues to contribute. Collaborations with other societies are discussed in section 2.1. An initial presentation for each chapter was given at early meetings of the group. Using comments made at the presentation, available literature as described above and the second edition of the Standards Document, a draft chapter was then produced and circulated. The authors guided the rest of the Subcommittee through the chapter at subsequent meetings, during which the evidence was evaluated. Following extensive discussion at these multidisciplinary meetings, a second draft was produced and any subsequent changes discussed at the next meeting. Where opinions differed, often because the evidence base was lacking, the group worked together to produce a form of words acceptable to the majority.

Standards and recommendations – definitions

1.6   We used the term 'standard' where the available evidence was strong or for key 'good practice' statements. In addition, it must be possible to audit a standard. We appreciate that not all the standards are subject to audit at present.

We used the term 'recommendation' where the available evidence was weaker and for other 'good practice' statements.

Peer review

1.7   The various chapters were then placed on internet sites used by patients and healthcare workers including, nurses, doctors (both adult and paediatric physicians), dialysis technicians, and dieticians. All members of the Renal Association and BAPN and all UK renal units received notification of the website addresses and contact was made with the Irish Society of Nephrology. In addition, a printed copy was sent to every renal unit in the UK for distribution to all interested staff members. One month was allowed for comment, and any received were forwarded to the chapter authors and to other members of the Subcommittee if appropriate. The draft document was discussed at a Plenary Session of the Renal Association in Spring 2001 and further helpful comments were received.

References

1   Cluzeau F, Littlejohns P, Grimshaw J, Feder G. *Appraisal instrument for clinical guidelines (version 1).* London: St George's Hospital Medical School, 1997.

2   US Department of Health & Human Services. Public Health Service and Agency for Health Care Policy & Research. *Acute pain management: operative or medical procedures and trauma.* Rockville, Maryland: Agency for Health Care Policy & Research (AHCPR publication 92-0038),1992.

2 | Epidemiology of chronic renal failure and renal replacement therapy

2.1   This chapter addresses the following questions:

▶   How common are chronic and end stage renal diseases (ESRD)?

▶   Who gets them?

▶   Does the incidence vary with place or time?

▶   What are the underlying causes?

▶   What is the need for renal replacement therapy (RRT) to treat ESRD?

▶   Is this being met?

▶   What is the survival rate on renal replacement therapy?

▶   How can we predict future demand?

Definition   2.2   End stage renal disease is the irreversible deterioration of renal function to a degree that is incompatible with life (in the absence of RRT, either by dialysis or transplantation), and is the end result of progressive chronic renal failure (CRF). The most valid measure of renal function is the glomerular filtration rate (GFR) which can only be measured by complex clearance studies (eg inulin). The clearance of the muscle breakdown product creatinine can be used, though at low levels of GFR creatinine clearance overestimates GFR (because of tubular secretion of creatinine, and extra-renal secretion into the gut). In practice, a patient is usually accepted as having ESRD when their creatinine clearance is <10 ml/min; in many patients this corresponds to a serum creatinine of about 500 µmol/l. Several factors influence creatinine production and clearance, such as age, sex, weight, ethnic origin, and muscle mass. A lower value of plasma creatinine may be indicative of ESRD in patients with low muscle mass (eg malnourished, or small Indo-Asian females). The Cockcroft and Gault formula uses age, sex, and weight and plasma creatinine to correct for these, and to estimate GFR. Whilst this formula is useful in clinical practice most epidemiological studies of CRF/ESRD have relied simply on measurement of serum creatinine.

2.3   The incidence of 'diagnosed' CRF in the population has been investigated in population-based studies using raised serum creatinine concentration obtained from chemical pathology laboratories. This is a specific, though insensitive, marker and it is usually measured as part of the urea and electrolytes test. This test is widely used to investigate patients who are unwell, to monitor those with chronic conditions such as diabetes, and as a pre-operative assessment of those requiring elective surgery. Such studies, therefore, exclude a proportion of people with CRF, such as those who are asymptomatic, who have not had a urea and electrolyte test, and/or high risk groups such as diabetics who have not had regular blood tests.[1] However, they are more likely to be representative than nephrology clinic studies where selection factors apply.[2]

2.4   Much of the information on the epidemiology of CRF has come from extrapolation from national acceptance rates for RRT. However, acceptance rates do not measure the incidence of ESRD as they are influenced also by levels of detection, referral and acceptance onto RRT. Moreover, it can be difficult to decide whether patients requiring dialysis who die in the early months had acute, acute on chronic, or chronic renal failure (see below).

2.5   Mortality data are unreliable because of significant under ascertainment[3] as are hospital episode statistics (HES) because they only relate to known treated cases who are admitted as inpatients; most RRT is delivered to outpatients or to patients at home. Moreover, International Classification of Diseases (ICD) coding does not reliably distinguish between acute and chronic forms of renal failure.

Population rates of CRF

2.6   Population studies of CRF have taken different cut-off values for serum creatinine concentration. Having a creatinine of over 500 µmol/l has been taken as evidence of ESRD, ie imminently needing RRT. Values lower than this are termed mild or moderate CRF (or pre ESRD), although this is a relative term as 60–70% of renal function is lost before serum creatinine concentration rises above the upper limit of normal (around 110–130 µmol/l). There have been two population-based studies of pre ESRD in the UK, both of which have used serum creatinine concentration as a marker of CRF:

i)   A study in the Grampian Region showed that the incidence of CRF (serum creatinine >300 µmol/l) was 450 per million population (pmp).[4]

ii)   A study using Southampton and South West Hampshire Health Authority as the population base found that in 1992–4 the annual incidence of newly diagnosed cases of CRF (serum creatinine >150 µmol/l) was 1700 pmp (95% CI 1562–1849).[5]

2.7   The incidence of ESRD in a given population determines the number of new cases that can be accepted for RRT. The prevalence of ESRD is almost the same as the prevalence of patients receiving RRT ('stock') because, if untreated, the survival of patients with ESRD is very short. The incidence of ESRD (based on routine serum creatinine concentration results over 500 µmol/l) has been defined by studies undertaken in Devon and the North-West by Feest et al,[6] and in Grampian by Khan et al.[4] These two studies gave similar results; the annual incidence of ESRD was 148 pmp per annum in the Feest study and 130 pmp in Khan's. There is a pyramidal relationship in population rates of 'diagnosed' CRF, the rates of moderate CRF being about three times greater than ESRD, and the rate of all known CRF over ten-fold more. The incidence of ESRD in a population will vary depending upon the population's age and sex distribution, ethnic composition, and according to indicators of social deprivation. These factors are discussed below.

CRF: age and gender

2.8   All the above studies show that CRF is predominantly a disease of the elderly, with rates rising almost exponentially with age. In the study from Southampton[5] the median age was 77; in Feest's study,[6] rates were 58, 160, 282, 503 and 588 pmp in the age groups 20–49, 50–59, 60–69, 70–79, and 80+ respectively. There is a male excess in all studies; in one study the ratio was 1:6.[5] This excess was only apparent over the age of 40 and it rose with age. Whilst the detailed gender breakdown was not published in Feest's and Khan's studies, re-analysis showed a male excess of 1.46; numbers within age groups were too small for reliable assessment (personal communication, Dr P Roderick, 2001). UK Renal

Registry data can at present only give ratios rather than rates. When full population coverage is achieved, age and sex rates can be calculated and assessment of the equity of provision by these factors can be undertaken.

CRF and ethnicity 2.9 Although there have been few population studies which have investigated the incidence of CRF and ESRD in ethnic groups, people of African or Afro-Caribbean origin and people of Indian sub-continent descent (Indo-Asians) are likely to have higher rates. In the USA, the acceptance rate of African Americans for RRT is four to five times higher than for whites and this is found for all causes except polycystic disease.[7] Direct extrapolation to African/Afro-Caribbean communities in the UK is not appropriate. There is, however, evidence that there is higher mortality from cerebrovascular and hypertensive disease[8] and a higher prevalence of hypertension among African/Afro-Caribbean populations than in whites in the UK.[9] The 1993 National Renal Review in England found that population-based ethnic-specific acceptance and stock rates in England were almost three times higher in African and Afro-Caribbeans than in whites and that the rate ratio increased with age.[10] The most common cause was diabetic ESRD.[11] People of Indo-Asian origin are known to have a higher prevalence and mortality from diabetes.[12] In the study carried out by the Southampton group, the small Indo-Asian population had a significant (2.5 fold) age adjusted increase in diagnosed CRF rate (>150 μmol/l) but numbers were small.[5] In the 1993 National Renal Review, Indo-Asians had increased rates similar to the African/Afro-Caribbean populations. These were even higher for diabetic patients with ESRD and for those whose ESRF had an uncertain cause.[10,11] In both ethnic groups there is evidence of more rapid progression of CRF to ESRD. This has been reviewed in a publication from the National Kidney Research Fund's 'a better life through education' (ABLE) project.[12]

2.10 The National Renal Review findings were confounded by inequality of access to renal services. Multi-level modelling of the data on the characteristics and location of all patients accepted onto RRT in England in 1991–2, demonstrated the independent effect of ethnicity (population levels of Indo-Asians and Afro-Caribbeans) on acceptance rates. After controlling for access to renal services, this provides indirect evidence of increased population need for RRT in these ethnic groups.[13] The increased acceptance rates amongst ethnic minority populations do not rule out inequality of access to services. Further population-based data are needed on the true incidence of CRF in ethnic minorities. Ethnic minority populations are much younger than whites. The implication is that as these populations age there will be an increased need, which will be disproportionate because of the age-related increases in relative rates. Age standardised acceptance rate ratios using the 1991–2 acceptance data were 90 pmp for whites, 422 for Asians and 374 for Afro-Caribbeans.[10] It has been estimated that the need for RRT in Greater London will grow by 25%-33% between 1991 and 2011 due to ageing of ethnic minorities and despite a net loss of the white population.[14] ESRD due to diabetes will be greater in districts with a high prevalence of people from ethnic minorities. A recent report estimated that because of increasing numbers of older people in ethnic minority groups between 1991 and 2011, the number of patients with diabetes will increase by 33.5% in Afro-Caribbean men, 79.4% in Afro-Caribbean women, 83% in Indo-Asian men and by 137% in Indo-Asian women.[15]

ESRD and socio-economic status

2.11 Another potentially important population determinant of the incidence of ESRD is socio-economic status. There are several types of evidence, though not all find an association:

i) There is a strong inverse social class gradient in mortality from renal failure.[16]

ii) The population-based rates of serum creatinine concentration over 150 µmol/l in Southampton and South West Hampshire increased in those areas with the highest Townsend deprivation index (a measure of the deprivation of an area based on census variables).[5]

iii) There is evidence for socio-economic gradients in underlying causes of ESRD such as Type 2 diabetes and hypertension.[17]

iv) Modelling studies of acceptances by area (ward level) deprivation show positive associations.[13,18]

v) Area deprivation was not found to be a factor associated with acceptance for RRT in two Scottish studies.[19,20]

Cause of CRF

2.12 It is difficult to ascertain the cause of ESRD from population-based surveys because most patients were not referred to nephrologists and had not received any definitive diagnosis. Most data come from studies of the causes of ESRD in patients accepted for RRT. This is a selected group which may under-represent certain causes, eg diabetes. Moreover as over 30% of patients requiring RRT present late, often with small shrunken kidneys, there is a high proportion where no obvious cause can be determined.[21] Furthermore there may be misclassification, especially in the categories of hypertensive ESRD, renovascular disease, and glomerulonephritis where no biopsy was performed. Diabetic ESRD was the commonest specific cause recorded in acceptance data at 19% in the 1998 Renal Survey, though data on type of diabetes are unreliable at present.[22]

Place and time variation in CRF

2.13 The incidence of CRF will be determined by the socio-demographic factors outlined above but there are no population data on such variation. There are no repeated surveys to address time trends; the only data come from acceptance rates. However, the rising acceptance rate in England (20 pmp in the early 1980s to over 90 pmp by 1998) does not imply that the incidence is rising[22] as this could at least in part be explained by an increased ability to treat ESRD. Nevertheless, there are factors which will increase the incidence: there is an epidemic of Type 2 diabetes[23] and an ageing population.[24]

What is the level of population need for RRT?

2.14 Feest *et al* estimated that the overall incidence of ESRD suitable for RRT in those aged less than 80 years old was 78 pmp per year (95% CI 63–93).[6] The 'suitability' criteria excluded patients who would have been likely to have had a severely restricted or hospital-based existence if accepted for treatment, eg those with severe vascular disease or advanced malignancy. In Feest's study 54% of incident cases of ESRD were referred for a nephrological opinion and 35% were accepted for treatment.

The need estimated was probably the minimum because:

▷ It did not take fully into account the needs of ethnic minorities.

▷ The over-80s were not included as they should have been, since chronological age is not a bar to treatment.

- Clinical thresholds for acceptance vary. In Wales and Scotland, and in several European countries where data are available for all patients with ESRD, acceptance rates in 1998 were over 100 pmp,[22,25] with Wales having a rate of 128 (115–140) pmp. If the Scottish age/sex acceptance rates are applied to the English population, with allowance made for the larger ethnic minority population in England and their greater rate of RRT, then the English acceptance rate would be about 115 pmp.

- The population is ageing; population estimates predict increases between 1994–2011 of 15% in the 60–74 age group and 14% in the over-75s.[24] This is particularly so for ethnic minorities as their currently relatively young population ages.

Standard

▶ While it is difficult to be precise about the level of national need for RRT, a realistic figure is an acceptance rate of at least 120–130 pmp. (B)

▶ It is likely that a minimum level of 100 pmp would apply to all health authorities/boards. (B)

2.15   At the primary care trust (PCT)/strategic health authority/board level the need for shared treatment will depend on the socio-demographic factors determining the incidence of ESRD, the most important being age and ethnic structure. Some areas with large ethnic minorities may have rates over 200 pmp, particularly as such populations age. The relatively small size of PCTs in England will mean that population rates will be subject to chance variation.

Is need being met?

2.16   The RRT acceptance rate for England rose through the 1990s from 67 (65–70) pmp in 1991/2 to 82 (80–85) pmp in 1995, and then to 92 (90–95) pmp in 1998.[22] In Scotland the rate was 105 (96–114) pmp in 1998, whereas Wales had a significantly higher rate of 128 (115–141) pmp. Significant regional variation in supply and acceptance rates persists.[22] These data suggest that population need is not being met either in England (particularly given the ethnic minority population), or to a lesser degree in Scotland. This unmet need is likely to occur in the older age groups and in patients with associated co-morbidity such as diabetes.

Measuring RRT rates

2.17   As with any epidemiological measure, we need to define 'acceptance'. This is difficult as there is no standard definition of the point at which a patient with ESRD enters the RRT programme, particularly if he/she presents as an uraemic emergency.[26]

Standard

▶ The Renal Registry definition of acceptance should be used in all units. (C)

2.18   A new patient with ESRD is here defined as:

▶   one who is accepted for treatment and transplanted or dialysed for more than 90 days

or

▶   one who is diagnosed as having ESRD (ie accepted for dialysis in the anticipation that they will need RRT indefinitely), dialysed, and dies within 90 days

or

▶   one who is dialysed initially for acute renal failure but is subsequently diagnosed as having ESRD.

Once a planned decision has been made, RRT is usually continued uninterrupted and the date of initiation is clear.[27] This excludes patients who were thought to have ESRD and started RRT in the expectation that this would continue indefinitely but who subsequently recovered within 90 days and are therefore classified in retrospect as having had acute renal failure.

2.19   Acceptance rates for RRT are dependent upon knowing the population base from which the data on new patients starting RRT are collected. This is possible if the postcode is known for all patients and the data from a given area are comprehensive; currently such data are available from Scotland and most of Wales. Rates of acceptance for RRT in England are based on estimated renal unit catchment areas from renal units. These are inevitably inaccurate though probably not systematically so, hence national rates may be reasonably valid.

2.20   Data on acceptance rates by health authority (HA) or health board (HB) will be available from the Renal Registry as greater population coverage in England is achieved and postcode data are mapped to HAs. Age, ethnic and gender rates by which to evaluate the equity of provision will also be available. In expressing rates, the age groups included should be stated. Most crude population rates are based on total populations, ie they include the population aged 0–15 in the denominator but may or not include the small number of childhood ESRD cases. Crude rates will be misleading as population age and ethnic structures vary.

Recommendation

▶ Each health authority/health board should assess its likely need for RRT in the light of the characteristics of the local population. These rates should be age and sex standardised and in future be standardised for ethnic minority populations, using 2002 Census data on health authority ethnic composition and Registry data on ethnicity. Such recording should be encouraged. (**Good statistical practice**)

Prevalent RRT rates

2.21   Prevalent cases are those currently receiving RRT; this group is also termed the 'stock' of patients. The prevalence rate will be the major factor determining the amount of provision and resource used in any given area. In simple terms it will reflect the pattern of acceptance over the preceding years, and the survival of patients once they have started on RRT. It is well recognised that units vary in the pattern of modalities of treatment provided to their prevalent stock. This will also occur once the prevalence rates for RRT are generated for the HAs by the Renal Registry. HAs/HBs can compare the balance of transplantation, haemodialysis and peritoneal dialysis with other areas in order to investigate to what extent these patterns are based on major resource constraints rather than clinical reasons and/or patient preference.

90-day rule   2.22   In the USA, for reimbursement purposes, patients are only regarded as starting the chronic RRT programme at 90 days following their first dialysis. The United States Renal Database System (USRDS), a major source of data on the largest RRT programme world-wide, reports all data from day 91 onwards. In several other countries patients with acute or CRF who die within the first 90 days may not be recorded as having ESRD.

Recommendation

▶ To allow meaningful comparison, UK performance should be analysed not only from the day of starting uninterrupted dialysis (day 0) but also from day 90. (**Good statistical practice**)

2.23   The first 90 days are, however, important since the highest rates of mortality, morbidity and costs arise during this period. It is important that patient numbers and the acceptance rate should be recorded from day 0. Inevitably there will be some grey cases presenting as uraemic emergencies who die without it being established whether there was underlying CRF or if they would have required long-term RRT. Application of the Registry definition attempts to standardise this between units.

Late referral   2.24   A major problem is that up to 40% of patients requiring RRT are only referred to the renal unit within four months of commencement of treatment.[28,29] This limits any prior care aimed at reducing cardiac risk or the complications of CRF, the opportunity to establish permanent access, to assess suitability for dialysis and allow patient choice of modality. Patients presenting as uraemic emergencies almost always start with emergency haemodialysis. Such patients are generally less well, having, for example, a lower albumin than those followed for longer; they have a stormier passage with longer hospitalisation and a higher mortality.[29] Detailed review of such cases has shown that a proportion of late referrals are unavoidable (eg late presenters with no prior symptoms or signs of CRF, or irreversible acute renal failure), but around 15% are potentially avoidable (Roderick, personal communication, 2001).

2.25   A recent audit of renal management in Scotland showed that 24% of patients who required dialysis for ESRD were known to a nephrologist, and had had a steady decline in renal function rather than an acute deterioration but none the less required an emergency first dialysis.[30] Such patients could have had access in place, and dialysis could have been planned. A further 12% had had an acute deterioration in renal function that could not have been predicted. Such unplanned emergency dialysis may thus be unavoidable, but should be audited.

▶ All renal units should audit late referrals to identify avoidable factors and any scope for improving the interface between primary and secondary care providers. (**Good practice**)

▶ Data should be provided to the Renal Registry at the time of first referral to the renal unit, and unplanned dialysis, so that the national pattern of late referral and its variation can be established. (**Good epidemiological practice**)

Analysing survival on RRT

2.26   As ESRD is universally fatal, survival is the ultimate outcome measure for patients starting RRT. It is influenced by a variety of factors. Some are fixed (eg age), others may not be under the direct influence of renal units (eg co-morbidity at start of RRT, albumin level at start of RRT), whilst others relate more directly to the quality of care (eg measures of dialysis adequacy). Hence, comparative audits of mortality within/between units and countries as a method of assessing the quality of renal care are misleading without adjustment for case mix. The age and co-morbidity of patients accepted onto RRT has changed dramatically over the last 20 years as referral and acceptance policies have become more liberal; currently nearly half of new patients are over 65 and nearly a fifth have ESRD resulting from diabetes.[22] It should be noted, however, that even when adjustment for co-morbidity and age is made, survival has been shown, in a retrospective study, to be lower in UK centres than in centres in France and Germany.[31]

2.27   Although data regarding age and gender are readily available, co-morbidity data are incomplete in the UK Renal Registry. Moreover, the optimal method of combining co-morbidity data is far from clear. The first National Renal Review simply used age and diabetes as cause of ESRD (though there are other patients with diabetes without diabetic ESRD).[32] The low-risk group were non-diabetics under 55; the medium-risk group were non-diabetics aged 55–64 and diabetics aged 15–54; and the high-risk group were non-diabetics aged 65 and above and diabetics aged 55 and above. The median survivals were 14.2, 7.4, and 3.5 years respectively. Khan *et al* developed an index combining age and presence of co-morbidity (coronary heart disease, heart failure, cancer, COPD/pulmonary fibrosis, liver disease) and diabetes which discriminated three groups as low, medium or high risk based on 2-year survival.[33] Such a mix of age and co-morbidity was found to be the most predictive in a comparison of different approaches.[34] However, with the changing profile of patients, many now fall into the high-risk category that may make this score insensitive to case mix differences. Moreover, heart failure can be difficult to classify. This suggests that co-morbidity should be assessed independently of age.

2.28   Chandra *et al* derived a predictive score based on age, a co-morbidity score, and Karnofsky performance status (a clinical assessment of the degree of dependency) that also discriminated three risk groups with significant survival differences.[35] There was only moderate overlap with the Khan Index. The co-morbidity score was complex, requiring assessment of the presence and severity of each condition (cardiac disease, peripheral vascular disease, cerebrovascular disease, respiratory disease, cirrhosis, cancer). Diabetes was modelled separately. The method of scoring was subjective, and the approach required validation in other patient cohorts prospectively. Unexpectedly, diabetes alone was not predictive, suggesting that the original age/diabetes classification is outdated. The Index of Coexisting Disease (ICED), which also has a weighted index of conditions and their severity, has been used in other conditions but not in renal patients in the UK.[36] Its use should probably be restricted to research rather than audit at this stage. The Renal Registry is trying to collect a detailed list of these conditions, since the limiting factor in any survival analyses is the quality of the co-morbidity information. A systematic quantitative review of the effect of co-morbidity on survival suggests that age, diabetes, heart disease and peripheral vascular disease are the major predictors of mortality.[37] It is important that we work out a minimum data set with good predictive powers to increase the feasibility of collection of co-morbidity data.

Recommendation

▶ All units registered with the Registry should endeavour to supply co-morbidity data on newly accepted patients. The priority should be diabetes as a cause of ESRD and evidence of coronary heart disease or peripheral vascular disease. (**Good practice**)

▶ Survival analyses must at least take account of age, gender, diabetes and co-morbidity. (**C**)

▶ The Karnofsky performance status is a simple measure that could be collected on incident and prevalent patients and used in survival analyses. (**B**)

2.29   Various measures of survival have been used. Survival from day 0–90 is an indication of the morbidity, particularly of those with unplanned or late referral. Such analysis is not possible in the USA because of the 90-day rule mentioned previously. One-year survival from the start of RRT is important for comparisons with non-US countries; for comparison with the USA one-year survival following day 90 is required. Prevalent one-year survival can be generated. With time the Registry will produce longer follow-up times, with 5-year survival. The annual mortality rates of incident/prevalent patients using person years as the denominator are informative, though it is important to note that prevalent patients are by definition survivors. The USRDS has used standardised mortality ratios whereby observed deaths in any unit are adjusted for by expected deaths, given the age, sex, ethnic and diabetes status of that unit's patients. A recent review of different methods of deriving SMRs showed how unstable they were over time, depending on the statistical method, the population included and the reference death rates. This was especially true for smaller units.[38]

2.30   It is hard to set survival standards at present because these should be appropriately grouped according to age, sex and co-morbidity and this is not yet possible from Registry data. The last Standards Document recommended at least 90% one-year survival for patients aged 18–55 with standard primary renal disease. This may have been too low as the rate in participating centres in the Registry was 97%, though numbers were small.

Planning for future demand

2.31   Commissioners and renal units will want to plan for future demand. A variety of models exist to try to predict this, varying from simple linear extrapolation of underlying trend in stock, through spreadsheet models to complex discrete event simulation based on individual patients.[39] No one model can be recommended, as it depends on the local expertise and data and resources available.

2.32   In most areas a steady state has not been reached at which input (acceptances per year and transfers in) is equal to the annual death rate and transfers out. Previous modelling suggested that this would not occur for over 20 years, so it is some way off.[39] The essential data required for modelling are:

i)   the inputs: current acceptance rate broken down by age, sex and if possible diabetes as a co-morbidity measure;

ii)   the current numbers of prevalent patients broken down in a similar way;

iii) the outputs: the simplest output would be annual mortality rates in the prevalent pool and in the first year on RRT (by age, sex and diabetes) giving an estimate of the additional patients added to the programme.

More sophisticated models can analyse the balance of modality using transplant survival and survival on the various modes of dialysis therapy. They can assess the availability and allocation of transplants and the amount of dialysis provision in a given area. Using the model, the acceptance rate can be increased to meet local need over varying time periods; the marginal effect diminishes as older and more co-morbid patients are added who have poorer survival. Patient survival can be varied.

Paediatric section

Incidence

2.33   The incidence of CRF (ie pre ESRD) in children is even more difficult to ascertain than in adults. Creatinine values of over 150 µmol/l are accepted as moderate CRF in childhood, but this figure is arbitrary because of the rising creatinine throughout childhood as muscle bulk increases. There have been a few studies of the incidence of CRF. However, comparisons are difficult due to different diagnostic definitions and different study populations. Over a period from 1972 to 1990, the incidence in reports from Germany,[40] Tunisia,[41] Sweden[42] and France[43] varied from 6 to 14.4 per million child population (pmcp) per year. In the epidemiological survey from France the prevalence of pre-terminal CRF in 1990 was 29 pmcp (<16 years), while the prevalence of ESRF was 37 pmcp. In the UK, a survey of nine comprehensive units in 1992 gave an estimated prevalence of pre-end stage CRF of 53 pmcp.[44] A variation in definition may be responsible for this significantly higher prevalence.

2.34   Information on ESRD in children in the UK has been obtained from data entered into the paediatric registry of the European Dialysis and Transplant Association,[45] surveys of the 13 UK-based Renal Units[44] and, more recently, from data collected through the National Paediatric Renal Registry.[46] These registries do not identify all patients, as they omit children who are not referred for ESRD management. Whilst this would be unusual, it may include an undocumented number of infants who are born with severe co-morbid conditions. At the other end of the spectrum, many new patients in the 15–18 years age group are referred directly to adult nephrology units. The quoted prevalence of ESRD in 1999 of 12.2 pmp or 53.4 pmcp may, therefore, be an underestimate. It is clear, however, that the number of patients under 18 years of age reported to the Registry has increased from 570 in 1992 to 755 in 1999. Of these, 429 were under 15 years of age in 1992 and 532 were under this age in 1999. This is an increase of 24% in the patient stock.

2.35   The take-on rate determined in 1999 in the under 14 years age group was 7.2 pmcp and in the under 18 years age group was 7.4 pmcp. The UK take-on rate documented in the European Dialysis and Transplant Association Report for 1989 was 5.2 pmcp in the under 15 years age group. Overall the average take-on rate in Europe at that time was 4.6 pmcp with about 7–8 pmcp in those countries with the most active treatment programmes. It is not clear whether a steady state has been reached yet.

Age and gender 2.36 As in adults, ESRD is more common in males than females, the male to female ratio being 1.76:1.[46] At a single audit point in 1999, the Paediatric Renal Registry documented 18 patients under 2 years of age and 311 in the 10–15 years age group, with a total of 532 patients under 15 years of age registered. There is a fall off in the 15–18 years age group (223 patients) reflecting different referral patterns and age of transfer to adult services.[46]

Ethnicity 2.37 In the 1999 Registry Report ethnicity data were available in 91% of the population. This showed an over-representation of Asians compared to that in the general population. The reasons are multifactorial and require further analysis.

Causes of ESRD 2.38 Diagnosis of the cause of ESRD is particularly important in paediatric practice because there may be genetic implications for the family. In the 1999 Registry report the commonest cause was renal dysplasia, occurring in 28% of patients (20% isolated renal dysplasia and 7.7% associated with other features). Obstructive uropathy accounted for 20.2% of cases (15.7% due to posterior urethral valves) and glomerulopathies accounted for 17%. Reflux nephropathy represented 7.2% of cases, which is less than previously reported. This is probably due to two reasons: firstly, an increased awareness of the significance of early treatment and investigation of urinary tract infection in childhood; and secondly, the realisation that many children who were previously classified as having reflux nephropathy have renal dysplasia. In a Chilean Survey from 1996,[47] 16.7% of patients had CRF or ESRD which was due to reflux nephropathy, whereas in Sweden, renowned for its active management of urinary tract infection in childhood, reflux nephropathy does not account for any patients with CRF or ESRD.[48]

Is need being met? 2.39 Many children are already in advanced CRF when first seen by a paediatric nephrologist. In the UK 1999 Registry data, more than a third were already in ESRD and a further 25% had GFRs of 10–20 ml/min/1.73 m^2. Only 13% had a GFR>50 when first seen. As most conditions are congenital or familial in origin, earlier referral should be possible. This is important if the adverse effects of CRF on growth and development are to be avoided. Kari[49] reported the outcome of 101 infants with CRF and found that with early enteral feeding the mean height standard deviation was within the normal range from one year of age, demonstrating the benefit of early intervention.

2.40 In recent years it has become possible to manage even infants with ESRD. However, this policy is not universally accepted, and management of these babies depends upon referral to a nephrology unit. Access to the service may therefore be restricted. The care of infants with ESRD is extremely labour intensive both for the medical team and the families. Many of these children have multiple problems in addition to the issues of growth and development. Management requires a full multidisciplinary team consisting of paediatric nephrologists, urologists, transplant surgeons and renal nurses, dieticians, psychologists, social workers, play specialists and teachers, to offer the comprehensive care that is needed. It is clear that the provision of these services is not uniform across the country, with some centres lacking the services that they need to provide comprehensive care. This is currently the subject of an extensive review of the provision of renal services across the UK.

References

1 Kissmeyer L, Kong C, Cohen J *et al*. Community nephrology: audit of screening for renal insufficiency in a high-risk population. *Nephrol Dial Transplant* 1999;**14**:2150–215.

2 Jungers P, Chauveau P, Descamps-Latscha B *et al*. Age and gender related incidence of chronic renal failure in a French urban area: a prospective epidemiological study. *Nephrol Dial Transplant* 1996;**11**:1542–6.

3 Goldacre MJ. Cause-specific mortality: understanding uncertain tips of the disease iceberg. *J Epidemiol Community Health* 1993;**47**:491–6.

4 Khan IH, Catto GRD, Edward N, MacLeod AM. Chronic renal failure; factors influencing nephrology referral. *Q J Med* 1994;**87**:559–64.

5 Drey N. *The epidemiology of diagnosed chronic renal failure in Southampton in South West Hampshire Health Authority*. PhD thesis. Southampton: University of Southampton, 2000.

6 Feest TG, Mistry CD, Grimes DS, Mallick NP. Incidence of advanced chronic renal failure and the need for end-stage renal replacement therapy. *BMJ* 1990;**301**:987–90.

7 United States Renal Data System. *1999 Annual Data Report. US Department of Health & Human Services, Public Health Service, National Institutes of Health*. Bethesda: National Institute of Diabetes and Digestive and Kidney Disease, 1999.

8 Balarajan R, Bulusu L. Mortality among migrants in England and Wales, 1978–83. In: Britten M (ed). *Mortality and geography: a review in the mid-1980s, England and Wales*. OPCS, Series DS no. 9, pp. 103–121 (see Appendix tables). London: HMSO, 1990.

9 Raleigh VS. Diabetes and hypertension in Britain's ethnic minorities: implications for the future of renal services. *BMJ* 1997;**314**:209–15.

10 Roderick PJ, Jones I, Raleigh VS, Mallick NP *et al*. Population need for renal replacement therapy in the Thames regions: the ethnic dimension. *BMJ* 1994;**309**:1111–4.

11 Roderick PJ, Raleigh VS, Hallam L, Mallick NP. The need and demand for renal replacement therapy in ethnic minorities in England. *J Epidemiol Community Health* 1996;**50**:334–9.

12 Lightstone L. *Preventing kidney disease: the ethnic challenge*. Peterborough: National Kidney Research Fund, 2001.

13 Roderick P, Clements S, Stone N *et al*. What determines geographical variation in rates of acceptances onto renal replacement therapy in England? *J Health Serv Res Policy* 1999;**4**:139–46.

14 Roderick P, Clements S, Diamond I *et al*. Estimating demand for renal replacement therapy in Greater London: the impact of demographic trends in ethnic minority populations. *Health Trends* 1998;**30**:46–50.

15 Gulliford MC, Melia A. Trends in diabetes mellitus in Greater London 1991-2011: associations with ethnicity. *Diabet Med* 1999;**16**:174–5.

16 Office for National Statistics. *Occupational health decennial supplement No. 10, 1995*. London: ONS, 1995.

17 Marmot MG, Davey Smith G, Stansfield S *et al*. Health inequalities among British civil servants: the Whitehall II study. *Lancet* 1991;**337**:1387–93.

18 Boyle OJ, Kudlac H, Williams AJ. Geographical variation in the referral of patients with chronic end-stage renal failure for renal replacement therapy. *Q J Med* 996;**89**:151–7.

19 Khan IH, Cheng J, Catto GRD *et al*. Social deprivation indices of patients on renal replacement therapy in Grampian. *Scott Med J* 1993;**38**:139–41.

20 Metcalfe W, MacLeod AM, Bennett D *et al*. Equity of renal replacement therapy utilisation: prospective population based study. *Q J Med* 1999;**92**:637–42.

21 Eadington DW. Delayed referral for dialysis. *Nephrol Dial Transplant* 1996;**11**:2124–6.

22 Feest T, Rajamahesh J, Taylor H, Roderick P. *The provision of renal replacement therapy for adults in the UK 1998*. London: Department of Health, September 2000.

23 Amos AF, McCarty DJ, Zimmet P. The rising global burden of diabetes and its complications: estimates and projections to the year 2010. *Diabet Med* 1997;**14**:S7–S85.

24 Government Actuary's Office. *National population projections 1994 based.* Series PP2 No 20. London: ONS, 1996.

25 Berthoux FC, Mehls O, Mendel S *et al.* Report on management of renal failure in Europe XXV 1994. *Nephrol Dial Transplant* 1996;**11**(Suppl 1):1–47.

26 Bhandari S, Turney JH. Survivors of acute renal failure who do not recover renal function. *Q J Med* 1996;**89**:415–421.

27 Hakim RM, Lazarus JM. Initiation of dialysis. *J Am Soc Nephrol* 1996;**6**:1319–28.

28 Obrador GT, Pereira BJG. Early referral to the nephrologist and timely initiation of renal replacement therapy: a paradigm shift in the management of patients with chronic renal failure. *Am J Kidney Dis* 1998;**31**:398–417.

29 Ellis PA, Reddy V, Bari N, Cairns HS. Late referral of end-stage renal failure. *Q J Med* 1998; **91**:727–32.

30 Metcalfe W, Khan IH, Prescott GJ *et al,* on behalf of the Scottish Renal Registry. Can we improve early mortality in patients receiving renal replacement therapy? *Kidney Int* 2000;**57**:2539–45.

31 Khan IH, Campbell M, Cantarovich D *et al.* Survival on renal replacement therapy in Europe; is there a centre effect? *Nephrol Dial Transplant* 1996;**11**:300–7.

32 Department of Health. *Review of renal services in England 1993–4.* London: NHS Executive, 1996.

33 Khan IH, Catto GRD, Edward N *et al.* Influence of coexisting disease on survival on renal replacement therapy. *Lancet* 1993;**341**:415–8.

34 Khan IH, Campbell MK, Cantarovich D *et al.* Comparing outcomes in renal replacement therapy: how should we correct for case-mix? *Am J Kidney Dis* 1998;**31**:473–8.

35 Chandra SM, Schulz J, Lawrence C *et al.* Is there a rationale for rationing chronic dialysis? A hospital based cohort study of factors affecting survival and morbidity. *BMJ* 1999;**318**:217–23.

36 Charleson M, Pompei P, Ales K *et al.* A new method of classifying prognostic comorbidity in longitudinal studies: development and validation. *J Chronic Dis* 1987;**40**:373–83.

37 Johnson JG, Gore SM, Firth J. The effect of age, diabetes and other co-morbidity on the survival of patients on dialysis: a systematic quantitative overview of the literature. *Nephrol Dial Transplant* 1999;**14**:2156–64.

38 Lacson E, Teng M, Lazarus JM *et al.* Limitations of the facility-specific standardised mortality ratio for profiling health care quality in dialysis. *Am J Kidney Dis* 2001;**37**:267–75.

39 Davies RM, Roderick P. Predicting the future demand for renal replacement therapy in England using simulation modelling. *Nephrol Dial Transplant* 1997;**12**:2512–6.

40 Pistor K, Scharer,K, Olbing H. Children with chronic renal failure in the Federal Republic of Germany I. Epidemiology. Modes of treatment, survival. *Clin Nephrol* 1985;**23**:272–7.

41 Tabbane C, Barsaoui S, Dliga Y, Arif M. L'insuffance renale chronique de l'enfant tunisien. *Tunis Med* 1986;**64**:1047–50.

42 Esbjorner E, Aronson S, Berg U *et al.* Children with chronic renal failure in Sweden 1978–1985. *Pediatr Nephrol* 1990;**4**:249–52.

43 Deleau J, Andre J-L, Briancon S, Musse J-P. Chronic renal failure in children: an epidemiological survey in Lorraine (France) 1975–1990. *Pediatr Nephrol* 1984;**8**:472–6.

44 British Association for Paediatric Nephrology. Report of a Working Party of the British Association for Paediatric Nephrology. *The provision of services in the United Kingdom for children and adolescents with renal disease.* London: BAPN, 1995.

45 Broyer M, Chantler C, Donckerwolcke R *et al.* The paediatric registry of the European Dialysis and Transplant Association: 20 years' experience. *Pediatr Nephrol* 1993;**7**:758–68.

46 Ansell D, Feest T (eds). The UK Renal Registry. *The second annual report*, 1999. Bristol: UK Renal Registry, 1999;175–87.

47 Lagomarsimo E, Valenzuela A, Cavagnaro F, Solar E. Chronic renal failure in Pediatrics. 1996 Chilean Survey. *Pediatr Nephrol* 1999;**13**:288–91.

48 Esbjorner E, Berg U, Hansson S. Epidemiology of chronic renal failure in children: a report from Sweden 1986–1994. *Pediatr Nephrol* 1997;**11**:438–42.

49 Kari JA, Gonzalez C, Lederman SE *et al.* Outcome and growth of infants with severe chronic renal failure. *Kidney Int* 2000;**57**:1681–7.

3 Haemodialysis – clinical standards and targets

Introduction

3.1　Haemodialysis (HD) remains the default therapy for all end stage renal disease (ESRD). Despite the success of transplantation and peritoneal dialysis (PD), HD continues to have the highest rate of growth of all treatment modalities.[1] Many patients are maintained by HD after rejecting transplants or because they have had to abandon PD. Furthermore, a number of PD patients transfer to HD during the last few months of their lives.[1] About 40% of patients starting renal replacement therapy (RRT) are referred as late uraemic emergencies with no time for the planning of, or counselling on, the options for dialysis,[2] and such patients are more likely to remain on HD.[3] These factors combine to increase the co-morbidity burden of the HD population. It is obvious that to improve survival on RRT requires that HD be delivered to a high standard.

3.2　HD treatment has evolved rapidly since its introduction, and continues to do so. Changes have seldom been underpinned by sufficiently large randomised trials. Nevertheless, day-to-day clinical decisions on appropriate treatments have to be made, and standards have to be set on the best available evidence.[4,5] HD may be performed in a variety of settings, including hospital-based units, free-standing units, and in the home. Not all UK units provide home HD. Where this option is available, the choice should be largely determined by patient preference rather than on economic grounds. Recently there has been an increase in some areas in the provision of home HD driven by the lack of space in hospital dialysis units. The standards set in this chapter apply equally to each of these settings.

Dialysis equipment and disposables*

Standards

▶ All equipment used in the delivery and monitoring of therapy should comply with the relevant standards for medical electrical equipment (BS-EN 60601-2-16:1998, BS 5724-2-16:1998, IEC 60601-2-16:1998. Medical electrical equipment. Particular requirements for safety. Particular requirements for the safety of haemodialysis, haemodiafiltration and haemofiltration equipment). (**Good practice**)

▶ Disposables such as dialysers and associated devices are classified as medical devices and should display the CE mark. The presence of such a mark signifies compliance with the national and international standards: haemodialysers, haemodiafilters, haemofilters, haemoconcentrators and their extra corporeal circuits (BS-EN 1283:1996). Plasma filters (BS/150 13960).

Recommendation

▶ Machines should be considered for replacement after seven years service or after completing 50,000 hours operation, whichever is first. (**Good practice**)

*See Appendix D for details of standards abbreviations used in this chapter.

RATIONALE

3.3   Equipment used in renal units represents a substantial asset which must be carefully maintained. The selection of equipment should be in accordance with a policy that conforms to the recommendations of the Medical Devices Agency (MDA) (Device Bulletin DB 9801, 1998, *Medical device and equipment management for hospital and community based organisations*) and National Audit Office (*The management of medical equipment in NHS acute trusts in England*, National Audit Office, 1999).

3.4   Renal units should endeavour to adopt a programme of phased replacement of older HD machines. Although it is possible to keep a dialysis machine operating safely for many years, practical considerations of obsolescence and maintenance costs require a more structured approach. When a particular model of a machine becomes obsolete, companies generally only undertake to supply replacement parts for seven years. We accept that there is no firm evidence that replacement, as suggested above, is the most cost-effective strategy.

Concentrates and water for dialysis

Standards

▶ Concentrates used, either purchased ready-made or manufactured 'in house', must meet the requirements of prEN 13867: 2002 (concentrates for HD and related therapies). (**Good practice**)

▶ Water used in preparation of dialysis fluid must meet the requirements of BS ISO 13959 2001 (water for HD and related therapies) for bacterial and chemical contaminants. If routine monitoring demonstrates continuous excess contamination, a phased programme to improve this should ensue. When alternatives to conventional HD with low flux membranes are used, such as haemodiafiltration and haemofiltration, more stringent limits in respect of bacterial contamination are mandatory. For such alternative applications microbial count should not exceed 0 Colony Forming Units (CFU)/ml and endotoxin level should be less than 0.015 IU/ml. (**Good practice**)

▶ A routine testing procedure for product and feed water should form part of the renal unit policy. Samples should be cultured on Tryptone Glucose Extract Agar or Reasoner's 2A and, for fungi and yeast, on malt extract agar or Sabourad's Dextrose Agar (all incubations at room temperature, ie 20–22°C). The frequency for testing should not fall below monthly and should be sufficiently frequent to detect trends. (**Good practice**)

RATIONALE

3.5   HD exposes the blood of the patient to in excess of 300 litres of water per week through a non-selective membrane, in contrast to an average 12 litres per week through a highly selective membrane (intestinal tract) in healthy individuals. Patient related applications require the production of water of appropriate chemical, bacteriological and microbiological purity. The combination of devices required to achieve this will be determined by the quality of the incoming water and how it is used in the renal unit or patient's home. Knowledge of the potentially harmful effects of trace elements and chemicals is still growing, and techniques of water treatment are continuously being developed. The Association for the Advancement of Medical Instrumentation (AAMI) in the USA has taken a useful lead in these areas over a number of years. These recommendations reflect the AAMI Standards and those of the European Dialysis and Transplant Nurses Association/European Renal Care Association (www.edtna-erca.org) (Appendix 1).

3.6   The dialysis membrane has long been regarded as an effective barrier against the passage of bacteria and endotoxin (potent pyrogenic materials arising from the outer layers of bacterial cells) from dialysis fluid to blood. This produced a complacent attitude towards the purity of dialysis fluid. About 10 years ago, several *in vitro* studies showed that intact membranes used in dialysers are permeable to bacterial contaminants.[6–8] The pore size of the membrane appears to be less important than the thickness and the capacity of the membrane to adsorb bacterial products. Consequently low flux (standard) dialysis does not necessarily translate into higher microbiological safety than high flux dialysis or HDF. Patients receiving standard dialysis treatment with low flux cellulose-based membranes (thickness 6–8 microns), may therefore be at greater risk of pyrogenic reactions (see below) than those treated using thicker synthetic membranes which have the capacity to adsorb endotoxins and endotoxin fragments. This increased adsorptive capacity arises from the hypophobic domains in the membrane structure, which bind such fragments by Van der Waals forces. In patients treated with high flux membranes, a risk of pyrogen transfer due to back filtration (a movement of dialysis fluid into the blood pathway of the device due to a pressure gradient rather than the diffusion gradient discussed above) may exist. Lonneman *et al*,[6] however, concluded that diffusion rather than convection is the predominant mechanism of trans-membrane transport of pyrogens, and back-filtration across pyrogen adsorbing membranes does not necessarily increase their passage. It should be emphasised that the adsorption capacity of the synthetic membranes is not infinite and that a breakthrough of pyrogenic substances can occur in the event of excessive water contamination.

3.7   Because a raised C-reactive protein (a sensitive marker of activation of the acute phase response) is associated with a significantly increased risk of death,[9–11] this has led to speculation that impure dialysate may contribute to an increased risk of death in dialysis patients. Impure dialysate has also been implicated in the pathogenesis of dialysis-related amyloidosis.[12–14] While this suggestion has not been tested in clinical practice, it would seem prudent to ensure that water is as pure as reasonably possible. A range of standards exist world wide in respect of microbiological purity of water used in RRT. Within the UK the current draft International Standard (ISO/DIS 13959) will be adopted as a British Standard (BS-EN 13959) and any water used in the preparation of dialysis fluid should meet the requirements of this standard as a *minimum*. The standard stipulates that the product water used in the preparation of dialysis fluid should have a total viable microbial count not exceeding 10^2 CFU/ml and an endotoxin content not exceeding 1 IU/ml (~0.25 ng/ml for the limulus amoebocyte lysate (LAL) test). Ultrapure water is readily achievable using modern water treatment techniques and should be regarded as the standard for all newly installed water treatment plants.[15]

Standard

▶ The dialysate should contain bicarbonate as the buffer. **(A)**

RATIONALE

3.8   One of the critical functions of dialysis is the correction of the metabolic acidosis caused by the diseased kidney's failure to excrete non-volatile acids and to regenerate bicarbonate. Bicarbonate is the natural buffer normally regenerated by the kidneys and was the initial choice as dialysate buffer. If, however, sodium bicarbonate is added to a calcium- or magnesium-containing dialysate, their respective carbonate salts will precipitate unless the dialysate is maintained at a low pH level. Since it does not precipitate calcium or magnesium, acetate was used as an alternative buffer[16] because of its rapid conversion to bicarbonate in the liver. In the late 1970s and early 1980s, a number of studies suggested that some of the morbidity associated with HD could be attributed to the acetate component of the dialysate.[17,18] This appears to have been unmasked by the introduction of high-efficiency and short-duration dialysis, using membranes with large surface areas. Acetate intolerance led to the reappraisal of bicarbonate as a dialysis buffer in the early 1980s and, following the solving of the issue of precipitation, to its reintroduction. A recent systematic review of 18 randomised trials indicated a reduction in the number of treatments complicated by headaches, nausea/ vomiting and symptomatic hypotension when bicarbonate was used.[19] Economic evaluations showed the cost of self-mix bicarbonate buffer to be similar to that of acetate. It should be noted, however, that even 'bicarbonate' dialysate contains moderate amounts of acetate.[20]

3.9   It is not possible to set evidence-based standards for other components of the dialysate. There is recent evidence, however, that dialysis of non-diabetic patients against glucose-free dialysate is associated with a surprisingly high rate of asymptomatic hypoglycaemia without an associated counter-regulatory response.[21,22] The long-term effects of repeated dialysis-induced hypoglycaemia are uncertain. Hypoglycaemia is not seen if the dialysate contains glucose, but glucose-containing dialysate is slightly more expensive.

Dialysis membranes

Standards

▶ Patients whose estimated life expectancy is more than seven years and who are unlikely to receive a transplant as a result of human major histocompatibility complex (HLA) sensitisation, high risk of recurrent disease, rare tissue type or other contra-indications (including personal choice), are at high risk of dialysis-related amyloidosis. Such patients, and those with symptoms of dialysis-related amyloidosis should, where possible, receive a dialysis regimen with better clearance of beta 2-microglobulin, and ultrapure dialysate. Such treatments include HD with high flux synthetic membranes and haemodiafiltration. **(B)**

▶ For other patients the balance of evidence favours the use of low flux synthetic and modified cellulose membranes over unmodified cellulose membranes. **(A)**

▶ Those reusing dialysers marked 'for single use only' should have read the MDA Device Bulletin DB 2000(04) *Single-use medical devices: implications and consequences of reuse.* **(Good practice)**

RATIONALE

3.10   The use of synthetic membranes which can have more porous characteristics (high flux) than standard cellulose membranes started in the mid-1980s with a view to increasing the depurative capacity of HD. Interest was heightened by the subsequent discovery that a number of these membranes (eg polysulphone, polyamide, polyacrylonitrile) had markedly less ability to activate complement and other cellular elements than standard cellulose, and hence decrease the inflammatory response, ie they were more bio-compatible.

3.11   Cellulose membranes have been modified to make them both more bio-compatible and of slightly higher flux (semi-synthetic membranes), and synthetic membranes with lower flux properties have also been produced. The cost of the latter two types of membrane is now approaching that of cellulose membranes although currently the high flux synthetic membranes cost about three times as much.

3.12   Dialysis-related amyloidosis is a disabling, progressive condition caused by the polymerisation within tendons, synovium, and other tissues, of β-2-microglobulin, a large (molecular weight (MW) 11,600) molecule which is released into the circulation as a result of normal cell turnover but is not excreted in renal failure and is not removed by cellulosic membranes. Exposure to bio-incompatible membranes may increase β-2-microglobulin generation.[15] Symptoms are typically first reported 7–10 years after commencing HD. A systematic review[23] of 27 randomised trials comparing cellulose, modified cellulose and synthetic membranes, showed a significant reduction in end of study β-2-microglobulin values when high flux synthetic membranes were used; one small study showed amyloid occurred less frequently with this treatment. High flux HD membranes remove β-2-microglobulin by a combination of diffusive clearance and adsorption; HDF removes substantially more as a result of convective clearance. Both treatments are thought to reduce the risk of developing dialysis-related amyloid.

3.13   Whether bio-compatible membranes have other advantages, as a result of the reduced activation of the inflammatory response during dialysis, is less certain. The systematic review showed no evidence of benefit when synthetic membranes were used compared with cellulose/modified cellulose membranes, in terms of reduced mortality or reduction in dialysis-related adverse symptoms.[23] Comparison of unmodified cellulose and modified cellulose membranes was not undertaken. Despite the relatively large number of randomised controlled trials (RCTs) undertaken in this area, none of the studies that were included in the review reported any measures of quality of life. Plasma triglyceride values were also lower with synthetic membranes in the single study that measured this outcome. Differences in these outcomes may have reflected the high flux of the synthetic membrane. Serum albumin was slightly higher at certain time points in some studies when synthetic membranes of both high and low flux were used. Given the adverse prognostic impact of hypoalbuminaemia in dialysis patients, this may be an important finding.[11,22,24–28] Further trials are needed, and several are in progress.

3.14   Adequate solute clearance can be achieved using higher blood and dialysis fluid flows, and higher surface area membranes, than in the past. Since small MW solute (eg urea) removal can be formally quantified by validated techniques, dialysis times can be reduced while maintaining 'equivalence' in the degree of blood purification. Since so-called 'middle molecules' (MW 200–20,000) diffuse only slowly into dialysis fluid, shortened treatment times have a proportionately greater deleterious effect on their clearance which may have implications for the long-term health of dialysis patients. Theoretically, reductions in sessional dialysis time can be more safely pursued if there is a concomitant improvement in middle molecular (MM) clearance, a goal which cannot be achieved by high blood flow rate or dialysis fluid flow rate and large surface areas of membranes impermeable to middle molecules. While the use of high flux membranes can increase this, a more effective way of promoting MM clearance is to superimpose convection upon standard diffusive blood purification technique using HDF. In this technique approximately 20 litres of 'extra' fluid, over and above the patients' interdialytic fluid gain, is removed through the dialyser and an equal volume of physiological 'replacement' fluid is returned to the blood downstream of the dialyser. HDF can be carried out safely and has been adopted as standard treatment in at least two UK centres.[29]

Re-using membranes

3.15 Haemodialysers and their extracorporeal circuits contain sterile non-pyrogenic pathways. Such items are generally marked for single use only, although some are now designed for multiple use in an individual patient. Reprocessing is a combination of processes aimed at cleaning, disinfection and sterilisation of the item. Within the UK, reprocessing of items marked 'for single use' is discussed in the Medical Devices Agency Device Bulletin DB 2000(04) *Single-use medical devices: implications and consequences of reuse*. This is obtainable from the Medical Devices Agency, Hannibal House, Elephant and Castle, London SE1 6TQ.

3.16 Re-use has been shown to be safe in a number of studies[30,31] and to have benefits, specifically the reduction in β-2-microglobulin. Some studies report an overall reduction in mortality among patients treated with re-used dialysers,[32] although this may depend on the type of membrane used and on the agent used for re-processing, the use of bleach being associated with lower mortality than use of formalin.[33,34] In this way high flux bio-compatible membranes can be used more cost effectively. In recognition of this, recently an agreement was reached between the Food and Drug Administration (FDA) in the USA and the manufacturers, requiring that some dialysers should be labelled 'for multiple use' and that manufacturers should issue protocols for the safe reprocessing of their devices. Currently, manufacturers have different marketing strategies in different countries and the main suppliers in the UK do not currently supply 'for multiple use' labels with the same devices which are so labelled in the USA. Eventually it is hoped that mass production will result in lower prices for high flux bio-compatible dialysers making them cost-effective without re-use.

Dialysis frequency and dose

Standards

▶ HD should take place at least three times per week in nearly all patients. Reduction of dialysis frequency to twice per week because of insufficient dialysis facilities is unacceptable. **(Good practice)**

▶ Every patient receiving thrice weekly HD should show:

either   urea reduction ratio (URR) consistently >65%

or   equilibrated *Kt/V* of >1.2 (calculated from pre- and post-dialysis urea values, duration of dialysis and weight loss during dialysis). **(B)**

Recommendations

▶ Patients receiving twice weekly dialysis for reasons of geography should receive a higher sessional dose of dialysis, with a total *Kt/V* urea (combined residual renal and haemodialysis) of >1.8. If this cannot be achieved, then it should be recognised that there is a compromise between the practicalities of dialysis and the patient's long-term health. **(Good practice)**

▶ Measurement of the 'dose' or 'adequacy' of HD should be performed monthly in all patients. All dialysis units should collect, and report to the Registry, data on pre- and post-dialysis urea values, duration of dialysis, and weight loss during dialysis. **(Good practice)**

▶ Post-dialysis blood samples should be collected either by the slow-flow method, the simplified stop-flow method, or the stop-dialysate-flow method (Appendix 2). The method used should remain consistent within renal units and should be reported to the Registry. **(B)**

RATIONALE

Frequency and duration

3.17   The most powerful determinant of solute removal is dialysis frequency rather than duration. The thrice weekly dialysis schedule has evolved from empirical considerations in the belief that it reconciles adequate treatment with adequate breaks between treatments to provide the patient with a reasonable quality of life, although there is no hard evidence for its superiority. Furthermore, all outcomes data have been derived from patient groups undergoing such dialysis schedules. The frequency of twice weekly dialysis has decreased world wide, including in the USA[35] where it fell from 12.9% to 3.6% of new patients between 1990 and 1996.

3.18   Only one, now outdated, US randomised trial where cellulose membranes and acetate dialysate were used, has addressed the issue of optimal dialysis time. The National Co-operative Dialysis Study randomised non-diabetic patients to one of four dialysis regimens, two with short (2.5–3.5 hour) and two with longer (4.5–5.0 hour) dialysis times, and two different time-averaged urea concentrations in each arm. Longer dialysis gave a better outcome.[36,37] A combination of economic constraints, better patient tolerance using improved machines and materials, and patient preference for shorter times[37] has resulted in a gradual reduction in the average length of dialysis sessions around the world. The mean time in the UK is 3 hours 46 minutes.

3.19   More recently, two approaches to more frequent dialysis sessions have been investigated. The first is dialysis for around two hours per day for six days, and the other a renewed interest in slow overnight treatment for 5–7 nights, which can deliver very large doses of dialysis and remove fluid such that anti-hypertensive treatment can be reduced to a minimum. Both regimes have been reported to give improved outcomes when compared with the more conventional regime of three sessions per week each of four hours.[38–42]

Dialysis adequacy   3.20   Dialysis adequacy is a global concept which includes clinical assessment of well-being, the impact on the patient's life and measures of the molecular clearance by the dialysis process. The molecular weights of the solvent and solutes to be cleared by dialysis range over three orders of magnitude, from small (water, urea) to large (β-2-microglobulin). Adequate clearance of the whole range of molecules by dialysis is important. For practical reasons haemodialysis adequacy is calculated using small, easily measured solutes such as urea.[43–5]

Three methods of assessing urea removal are in current use:[43–4]

1   The URR[46] is the simplest. The percentage fall in blood urea effected by a dialysis session is measured as follows:
{(pre-dialysis [urea] – post-dialysis [urea])}/pre-dialysis (urea) × 100%.

2   *Kt/V* urea can also be predicted from one of several simple formulae requiring as input data the pre- and post-dialysis urea concentrations, the duration of dialysis, and the weight loss during dialysis.

3   Urea kinetic modelling (UKM) involves analysis of the fall in (urea) during haemodialysis, the rise in (urea) in the interdialytic period, clearance of urea by residual renal function, and the total clearance predicted from the dialyser clearance, blood and dialysate flow, time on dialysis, and fluid removal during dialysis. These data are fed into a computer programme which, assuming steady state, calculates *Kt/V* urea and normalised protein catabolic rate.[47]

All these methods require accurate measurement of pre-dialysis and post-dialysis urea concentrations on a mid-week dialysis session. Full urea kinetic modelling also requires:

▶   measurement of dialyser clearance

▶   measurement of weight loss during dialysis

▶   collection of an inter-dialytic urine for measurement of urea concentration and volume

▶   a pre-dialysis blood urea concentration from the subsequent dialysis session.

3.21   The URR does not take convective removal of urea into account, and therefore tends to underestimate the 'dose' of dialysis. Its accuracy is less than *Kt/V* measured by formal UKM, particularly at high values of URR and *Kt/V*.[48] URR does not take residual renal function into account, hence adjustment of dialysis dose to achieve a particular target will result in higher overall urea removal than anticipated in those with residual renal function. Despite these drawbacks, a number of observational studies in populations of dialysis patients have shown that variations in URR are associated with major differences in mortality.[28,49–51]

3.22   *Kt/V* can be calculated using several formulae giving different results[52] and hence for comparative audit it is important that the raw data are collected to allow calculation of URR and estimated *Kt/V* using a single formula.

3.23   Formal UKM, the most complex measure, requires collection of additional data on dialyser clearance, an interdialytic urine collection, and measurement of pre-dialysis urea concentration on the subsequent dialysis. Widely available computer software is required to perform the calculations. Its major advantage is that it allows much more accurate prediction of the effects of changing one particular component of the dialysis prescription (eg dialyser size, dialysis duration, blood-flow) on the delivered dialysis dose. UKM also gives valuable information on urea generation rate and protein catabolic rate. If the patient is in a steady state nutritionally, this gives information on current protein intake, and is a useful adjunct to other methods of assessment of nutritional status.

3.24   Many UK renal units only collect pre- and post-dialysis urea concentration, and only a very few perform UKM.[1] For comparative audit, the choice therefore currently lies between calculation of URR and estimation of Kt/V urea from such data. This situation is likely to change if more units adopt formal UKM. A retrospective analysis suggested that a Kt/V of 1.0 was the watershed between 'good' dialysis (>1.0), and inadequate dialysis (<1.0). Thereafter Kt/V survived as a recognised index of dialysis adequacy.[53] The remaining data relating dialysis dose to outcome are observational. Early studies showed that risk of death is associated with short dialysis duration[54] and low urea reduction ratio.[28] More recent studies[49–51,54–6] have shown a reduced mortality, with increasing dialysis dose measured in various ways; in some of these studies adjustment was made for co-morbidity.[51,57]

3.25   The optimal dialysis dose has not yet been defined. One study showed no further reduction in mortality above Kt/V of 1.3 or URR of 70%.[50] Many commentators, however, believe that there is some further improvement in mortality risk with Kt/Vs of up to 1.6 or even higher.[58–61] For the present we have retained our standard as Kt/V of 1.2 which should be regarded as a minimum requirement. The HEMO trial is a prospective randomised controlled trial in which patients have been randomised to an equilibrated Kt/V of 1.0 or 1.4 and to synthetic or semi-synthetic membranes of high or low flux.[62] Its results are expected soon. As with all standards, achievement is dependent on patients' adherence to treatment, for instance willingness to dialyse three times a week for the requisite number of hours. Increasing understanding amongst patients of the benefits of adequate dialysis should help further to improve outcomes.

Post-dialysis sampling

3.26   All measurements of dialysis dose require measurement of the post-dialysis blood urea concentration. Contamination of the post-dialysis sample with blood returning from the dialyser or heparin, or sampling from a fistula or other access device in which there is recirculation of dialysed blood will lead to falsely low measurements, and thus to over-estimation of dialysis dose. True venous blood urea concentration rises rapidly in the first few minutes after dialysis has ceased. It continues to rise at a rate higher than that expected from urea generation for up to 30 minutes, as a consequence of continued transfer of urea from peripheral body compartments into the bloodstream;[63–7] the earlier the sample is drawn, the higher the apparent delivered dialysis dose. Small variations in the timing and technique with which post-dialysis blood samples are drawn can, therefore, result in clinically important errors in the estimated dose of dialysis. Such variation has been shown to be common in the USA[68] and in the UK.[1] This suggests that changes, over time, in the technique for post-dialysis sampling causing higher apparent URR, have been responsible for an apparent rise in the URR necessary for optimum survival.[69] Several methods of standardisation of post-dialysis sampling are in use in the UK. The slow-flow method and the stop-flow method (Appendix 2) were devised to give immediate post-dialysis measurements while avoiding the effects of re-circulation within the fistula. Currently used formulae to predict 'equilibrated' blood urea have been validated using similar sampling methods. The stop-dialysate-flow method allows more re-equilibration and therefore results in systematically higher measurements of post-dialysis blood urea concentration.[70] This is currently the most widely used method in the UK.[1]

3.27 A post-dialysis rebound in venous blood urea concentration results from continued return of blood from poorly dialysed body 'compartments', and is particularly marked after high efficiency dialysis. Accurate comparison of delivered dialysis dose therefore requires estimation of the equilibrated blood urea concentration, allowing calculation of 'equilibrated' Kt/V. Full re-equilibration takes about 30 minutes, but it is impractical to ask patients to wait this long for post-dialysis blood sampling on a routine basis. The amount of rebound is determined by several factors including the intensity of dialysis and the size of the patient. Several formulae, which predict the equilibrated post-dialysis urea concentration, have been validated. The three formulae in widespread use in the UK – the Smye, Daugirdas, and Tattersall equations – give very similar results.[67] All of these formulae have been validated using an immediate post-dialysis sample; prediction of equilibrated dialysis dose using the stop-dialysate-flow method requires a different formula.[71]

Dialysis-related hypotension

Recommendation

▶ Data on the frequency of dialysis-related hypotension, defined as an acute symptomatic fall in blood pressure during dialysis requiring immediate intervention to prevent syncope, should be collected and reported to the Renal Registry. (**Good practice**)

RATIONALE

3.28 Dialysis-related hypotension is the most frequent symptom to complicate dialysis and can be extremely unpleasant, as well as reducing the efficiency of dialysis.[72] The frequency of this event is, therefore, an important indicator of the quality of dialysis from the patient's perspective. It is caused by a reflex withdrawal of sympathetic tone resulting from decreased left ventricular filling, and is therefore dependent on the rate of fluid removal from the vascular space, the rate of re-filling from the interstitial space, venous tone, and many other variables.[73] Patients experiencing frequent dialysis-related hypotension are at higher risk of death,[74] although this may be because dialysis-related hypotension is a marker for severe cardiac disease[75]. Adjustment of the rate of fluid removal, dialysate sodium concentration, and dialysate temperature during dialysis, can reduce the incidence of this complication,[72,76] but incurs an increased cost due to the need for on-line monitoring of changes in relative blood volume (by measurement of changes in optical density of blood).

▶ At least 67% of patients presenting within three months of dialysis should start HD with a usable native arteriovenous fistula. (**Good practice**)

▶ At least 80% of prevalent HD patients should be dialysed using a native arteriovenous fistula. (**Good practice**)

▶ No patient already requiring dialysis should wait more than four weeks for fistula construction including those who present late. (**Good practice**)

▶ All dialysis units should collect data on infections related to dialysis catheters and polytetrafluoroethylene (PTFE) grafts to allow internal audit. (**Good practice**)

RATIONALE

3.29   The preferred access in the great majority of HD patients is a native arteriovenous fistula (AVF) which produces the highest flows, minimises sepsis and has the greatest longevity. Although most AVFs are created at the wrist, not all are successful and, while some patients go on to have AVFs created at the elbow, about 20% will be dependent upon intravenous plastic cannulae tunnelled under the skin or grafts made of synthetic tubing inserted under the skin. In a small number, severe cardiac dysfunction is seen as a contra-indication to fistula construction, as a high flow AVF can contribute to high output cardiac failure.

3.30   In practice, fewer patients have AVFs for two main reasons. Firstly, up to 45% of patients starting HD do so as uraemic emergencies where there has been no time to create permanent access.[77] Secondly, most renal units in the UK have insufficient access to surgical support including theatre sessions dedicated to renal failure surgery. Temporary and semi-permanent tunnelled catheters are unfortunate necessities for many patients awaiting creation of a natural AVF; once established on dialysis via a catheter, some patients may, despite counselling, refuse to have an AVF constructed.[78] The high numbers of patients with temporary and tunnelled lines generally indicate congestion in a service with inadequate surgical support. Use of dialysis catheters and PTFE grafts for dialysis is associated with a greatly increased risk of hospitalisation and sepsis than use of AVFs.[79,80]

3.31   The UK is therefore lagging behind most of the larger countries with regard to the proportion of HD patients using natural AVFs. Data from the Dialysis Outcomes and Practice Patterns Study (DOPPS) show that 67% of prevalent patients in the UK have functioning AVFs, compared with the European average of 80%. This study includes data from the UK, France, Germany, Italy and Spain. Only 47% of UK patients start with a functioning AVF, compared with a European average of 66%.[81]

Paediatric section

3.32 Pre-emptive transplantation is usually considered for children in whom there is a predictable decline in renal function to ESRD. When dialysis is required, PD is the first choice in most paediatric units, with a ratio of PD to HD of 2:1 in the UK[82] and North America,[83,84] although this proportion becomes equal by adolescence. There is no evidence that PD is superior to HD, but in most instances HD is more disruptive to family life and schooling. It is usually reserved for children who are unable, for physical or social reasons, to be managed by PD at home.[84] However, experience dictates that a paediatric dialysis programme should be able to provide both in-centre HD as well as home and in-centre PD. It is more usual for patients to be transferred from PD to HD because of complications rather than vice versa. The length of time on HD is usually short because of the shorter waiting times for transplantation in children. The relatively smaller numbers of paediatric patients means that there are few controlled comparative studies in children. Guidelines are based on opinions and reports of clinical experience to registries.

The dialysis centre

Standard

▶ All children requiring HD should be treated in a designated paediatric nephrology and dialysis centre. (**Good practice**)

Recommendations

▶ Children and parents should be free to choose a particular dialysis modality in discussion with the multi-professional team.[85] (**Good practice**)

▶ It is essential that children receiving chronic HD treatment are given a service that meets their physical and psychosocial needs. Children should be nursed in paediatric units where a renally trained children's nurse is always available for advice and support.[86] (**Good practice**)

▶ The child and family should be prepared either in hospital or at home for HD by their named nurse and play specialist using such materials as dolls, videos, story books and games.[87] (**Good practice**)

▶ The child's nutritional status should be managed and monitored by a paediatric renal dietician. (**Good practice**)

Vascular access

Standards

▶ Temporary central venous lines risk the loss of potential access points and their use should be kept to a minimum. (**Good practice**)

▶ When tunnelled, cuffed central venous catheters are used, the rate of infection should be better than one in every 12 patient months averaged over the total population for three years.[88] (**Good practice**)

▶ The choice of vascular access should take into account the age and size of the child. Although an arteriovenous fistula is regarded as the best long-term vascular access, this may not be possible in small children who can be managed using catheters that are tunnelled subcutaneously. Such catheters can also provide vascular access in older children where early transplantation is anticipated. (**Good practice**)

▶ Vascular access should be performed by an appropriately trained surgeon. (**Good practice**)

▶ Problems with needle phobia require referral to a child psychologist. (**Good practice**)

Dialysis frequency and dose

Standards

▶ Standards of adequacy recommended for adult patients should be regarded as the minimum for children. (**Good practice**)

▶ Adequacy tests should be performed monthly. (**Good practice**)

RATIONALE

3.33   In view of the lack of paediatric evidence, it is recommended that adult values for measures of small solute clearance, *Kt/V*, creatinine clearance and urea reduction ratio are extrapolated to children. It is worth stressing that in paediatric practice, as with adults, adequate dialysis is a combination of a number of factors and not just small solute clearance. If assessing urea reduction ratio, then this should occur at least monthly and may need to take place at least once every two weeks in young children. Residual renal function should be measured three monthly in children able to provide 24-hour urine collections. The HD prescription needs to be adjusted in line with growth and changing nutritional requirements.

3.34   Post-dialysis target weight should be reassessed monthly in order to allow for growth. Patients with regular weight gains of >6% of post-dialysis target weight should be identified and given help to achieve fluid control.

3.35   Untoward complications are prevented by thorough assessment and monitoring before, during and after HD of weight, blood pressure, temperature, pulse, general well-being and fluid assessment.

3.36   The extracorporeal blood volume in the HD circuit is recommended not to exceed 8–10% of the child's total blood volume (80 ml/kg).[89] All children should be dialysed with a machine offering volume controlled ultrafiltration and should receive bicarbonate dialysis using a bio-compatible dialyser. When choosing a dialyser, the urea clearance is estimated at 3–5 ml/kg/min where the effective surface area of the dialyser is less than three-quarters of the child's body surface area.[90]

3.37   URR is a mathematically simple, transparent and easily applied measure of small solute clearances. It avoids assumptions required to perform more complex formal UKM.[91]

However, URR underestimates true urea clearance, as it does not measure urea removed by native kidney function and ultrafiltration. The greater the urine clearance, the greater the underestimate. It is likely in the near future that direct measurement on-line of urea removal will be available, thus removing the need for mathematical modelling. In children with no, or unmeasured, residual renal function, URR should be equal to or more than 65%. Children with residual renal function may be well dialysed with URR <65%.

3.38 The guideline for removing fluid in dialysis is no greater than 5% post-dialysis target weight per session (0.2ml/kg/min).[89] Weight gain between dialysis treatments should be recorded for each dialysis session, and should be encouraged to be 5% or less between sessions, often requiring a fluid restriction. For more fluid removal during the session, isolated ultrafiltration at the beginning of treatment may reduce symptoms.

Psychosocial support (for HD and PD)

Standard

▶ Psychosocial support is an essential part of the care offered to children and families while on dialysis. All members of the multidisciplinary team contribute to such support, but the social worker and psychologist will play lead roles. (**Good practice**)

Recommendations

▶ Each paediatric unit should have a suitably qualified and experienced social worker allocated to the work of the unit and involved in arranging appropriate information and support for each family. In addition, the social worker should assess the economic impact of dialysis on the family and discuss possible sources of financial support. (**Good practice**)

▶ Dialysis, particularly in infants, imposes a large burden of care upon families. Strategies such as home-care nursing, respite care and holidays for children need to be considered to prevent family burn-out.[92] (**Good practice**)

▶ Children attending the HD unit on a regular basis have the greatest need for educational support as they will miss considerable school time. Liaison between the hospital school-teacher and the child's school is essential for all hospitalised children.[93] (**Good practice**)

▶ Adolescent patients will require an additional profile of education plans, social issues and careers advice. The timing and practicalities of transition to adult units have to be actively discussed and planned.[94] (**Good practice**)

Research and audit

▶ Each paediatric renal unit should maintain mortality and morbidity data for patients on HD. All vascular access related problems, such as catheter malfunction, exit site and tunnel infections, septicaemia rates, results of dialysis adequacy parameters and their relationship to growth, should be maintained by each unit. The data should be reported to the British Paediatric Renal Registry to be used for comparative audit and setting of standards. (**Good epidemiological practice**)

Access to and withdrawal from dialysis

Recommendation

▶ The decisions to institute active non-dialytic management of the patient with ESRD, including nutritional, medical and psychological support, or to discontinue dialysis already in train, should be made jointly by the patient and the responsible consultant nephrologist after consultation with relatives, the family practitioner and members of the caring team, abiding by the principles outlined briefly below. The decision, and the reasons for it, must be recorded in the patient's notes. The numbers of patients not taken on to dialysis and the reasons for this decision should be subject to audit, as should the numbers and causes for those in whom dialysis is discontinued. Centres should develop guidelines for palliative care of such patients, including liaison with community services. (**Good practice**)

RATIONALE

3.39   Now that every patient in chronic renal failure, of whatever age and co-morbidity, is at least considered as a potential recipient of dialysis, questions of deciding not to start or to terminate dialysis have assumed increasing importance. Until recently, the UK dialysis scene was characterised by accidental – but also sometimes deliberate – failure of referral, so that the decision not to treat was taken by family members or referring physicians alone, rather than in conjunction with a nephrologist,[95] and there have been few studies of the decision not to start dialysis.[96–7] Equally, there is only one study from the UK of withdrawal from dialysis[98] suggesting that this plays a major role (17%) in overall death rates on dialysis, as it does in the USA and Canada.[99–101]

3.40   In practice, the decision not to take a patient on to dialysis has much in common with the decision to withdraw dialysis. This is because caring staff, patients and relatives, all face similar difficult[102] judgements and decisions about the likely quality and quantity of life on dialysis. Also, two approaches may be taken when a patient presents in uraemia whose ability to cope with, and to enjoy and benefit from, dialytic treatment is doubtful. The first approach attempts to make a 'clean' decision on whether or not to start dialysis after a process of consultation and discussion; the second, often called 'trial of dialysis', involves starting a proportion of such patients on dialysis, but with a pre-discussed plan to review whether this should continue beyond a specified point in the near future – usually a few weeks or months. Clearly the expectation is that the outcome in this case will be withdrawal of some patients from dialysis.

3.41   In addition to patients who clearly present greater than average problems from the outset, there are individuals who have had a period of worthwhile life on dialysis, but whose quality of life worsens because of medical or psychological deterioration, or both simultaneously. Additional difficulty arises when dementia, often fluctuating, makes it hard or impossible to ascertain what the patient's own feelings and wishes might be.

3.42   It is impossible to set quantitative standards in this difficult area of care, but principles of action can be enunciated and agreed. All patients in renal failure should be considered for dialysis, and neither age *per se* nor the social situation and support (or lack of it) should be a factor leading to exclusion. Nor should lack of facilities for dialysis be acceptable on its own as grounds for exclusion, or fear of litigation a basis for a decision in either direction.

3.43 Careful medical assessment of any co-morbid conditions from which the patient may suffer is needed, together with whatever medical measures (short of dialysis) are required to correct them or minimise their effects.[103] Particular attention needs to be paid to potentially reversible mental states. Similarly, patients who have deteriorated will need careful medical and psychological assessment. If it appears that only a brief period of survival of unacceptable quality is likely on dialysis (eg less than three months), then the possibility of not starting or stopping dialysis needs to be considered. The interest of the individual patient must remain paramount, and although the opinions of relatives should be consulted, they should not be binding. The responsible consultant nephrologist should solicit views of the patient's family doctor, next of kin, and all carers within the multidisciplinary caring team. The decision must be taken by both the consultant (who must assess the patient personally), and the patient. The patient will need to be fully informed throughout, and to be aware of their options, so far as their mental status permits. The most realistic and accurate description of starting or not starting, continuing or not continuing dialysis should be given. The substance of these discussions must be recorded in the patient's notes. If the decision is taken not to initiate, or to stop dialysis, then a management plan of supportive care must be put in place. This must then be carried through in a way that ensures continued support, achieves what seems best *from the patient's point of view,* and finally enables the patient to die with dignity, when the time comes. Achieving this will often require co-ordinated work with the palliative care team, who should be involved early in the management plan.[104] Certain patients who are severely ill, often with conditions affecting several organs, may have a concurrent acute deterioration of their chronic renal failure. The referring physician (who may be in a different hospital) and the nephrologist, may feel, after discussion, that dialysis is inappropriate given the very poor prognosis from the underlying conditions. Under these circumstances the referring physician would discuss matters with the patient, if possible, and with the family.[97]

Paediatric section

3.44 In paediatric practice, in particular, the decision to focus on palliative care often evolves gradually. Different members of staff and family may be working towards the decision at different rates, and time and discussion are essential for the transition. This time can be helpful in providing an opportunity for planning, as medical, nursing, psychosocial and spiritual care needs to be provided.

Recommendations

▶ Centres should have guidelines for palliative care.

▶ Symptom management should include assessment of current problems as well as prediction of future ones, and a management plan should be prepared.

▶ Plans for any equipment necessary should be made before it is needed.

▶ Possible drug requirements and their routes of administration should be predicted.

▶ Community nursing support should be arranged.

▶ Access to 24-hour support should be arranged. A key worker, usually a hospital or community nurse, should take on the task of coordinating care.

▶ Information should be provided as to how the child may die and what to do after death.

▶ Support should be available for the child to discuss their illness if they are old enough, and should be available for siblings and other family members.

Appendix 1

Specification for chemical analysis of treated water for dialysis

(Based on AAMI standards[105] but modified in accordance with current British and European Pharmacopoeias)

1. pH	5.0–7.0	10. Calcium	Limit 2 ppm
2. Chlorine	Limit 0.1 ppm/mg/l*	11. Magnesium	Limit 2 ppm
3. Chloramine	Limit 0.1 ppm	12. Copper	Limit 0.1 ppm
4. Chlorides	Limit 50 ppm	13. Zinc	Limit 0.1 ppm
5. Nitrate	Limit 2 ppm	14. Lead	Limit 0.005 ppm
6. Sulphate	Limit 50 ppm	15. Mercury	Limit 0.001 ppm
7. Fluoride	Limit 0.2 ppm	16. Silver	Limit 0.005 ppm
8. Sodium	Limit 50 ppm	17. Aluminium	Limit 0.01 ppm
9. Potassium	Limit 2 ppm	18. Ammonium	Limit 0.2 ppm

* The units ppm and mg/l are equivalent

Appendix 2

Methods for post-dialysis sampling

Slow-flow method

Guidelines developed by F Gotch and M Keen, Davis Medical Centre, San Francisco and used since 1990 by Lister Renal Unit, East & North Herts NHS Trust.[64]

▶ At the end of dialysis, turn the blood pump down to 100 ml per min.

▶ Override alarms to keep blood flowing.

▶ Wait 15–30 seconds and take samples from the 'A' line sampling post.

▶ If more than one sample is required, the urea should be the first one taken.

▶ Wash back blood; take patient off as normal.

Simplified stop-flow method

Guidelines developed by EJ Lindley, V Osborne, S Sanasy, D Swales and M Wright. The Leeds Teaching Hospitals NHS Trust.

▶ When you are ready to take the sample, turn the blood pump slowly down to 50 ml/min.

▶ Start counting to five; if the venous pressure alarm has not already stopped the blood pump when you get to five, stop the pump manually.

▶ Disconnect the arterial line and take a sample from the needle tubing (or the arterial connector of the catheter) within 20 seconds of slowing the blood pump to 50 ml/min.

▶ If more than one sample is required, the urea sample should be the first one taken.

▶ Wash back blood; take patient off as normal.

Stop-dialysate-flow method

Developed by Dr Mactier, Geddes, and Traynor at Stobhill Hospital Glasgow, and now currently used by all dialysis units in Scotland.[70]

▶ Stop dialysate flow, but keep blood pump running for five minutes.

▶ Take a blood sample from anywhere in the blood circuit.

References

1   Ansell D, Feest T (eds). UK Renal Registry. *The third annual report*, 2000. Bristol: UK Renal Registry, 2000.

2   Metcalfe W, Khan IH, Prescott GJ *et al*. Can we improve early mortality in patients receiving renal replacement therapy? *Kidney Int* 2000;**57**(6):2539–45.

3   Little J, Irwin A, Marshall T *et al*. Predicting a patient's choice of dialysis modality: experience in a United Kingdom renal department. *Am J Kidney Dis* 2001;**37**(5):981–6.

4   Wolfe RA. Observational studies are just as effective as randomized clinical trials. *Blood Purif* 2000;**18**(4):323–6.

5   Greene T. Are observational studies 'just as effective' as randomized clinical trials? *Blood Purif* 2000;**18**(4):317–22.

6   Lonnemann G, Behme TC, Lenzner B *et al*. Permeability of dialyzer membranes to TNF alpha-inducing substances derived from water bacteria. *Kidney Int* 1992;**42**(1):61–8.

7   Evans RC, Holmes CJ. *In vitro* study of the transfer of cytokine inducing substances across selected high flux hemodialysis membranes. *Blood Purif* 1991;**9**:92–101.

8   Laude-Sharp M, Caroff M, Simard L *et al*. Induction of IL-1 during hemodialysis: transmembrane passage of intact endotoxins (LPS). *Kidney Int* 1990;**38**(6):1089–94.

9   Owen WF, Lowrie EG. C-reactive protein as an outcome predictor for maintenance hemodialysis patients. *Kidney Int* 1998;**54**:627–36.

10 Zimmermann J, Herrlinger S, Pruy A *et al*. Inflammation enhances cardiovascular risk and mortality in hemodialysis patients. *Kidney Int* 1999;**55**:648–58.

11 Ikizler TA, Wingard RL, Harvell J *et al*. Association of morbidity with markers of nutrition and inflammation in chronic hemodialysis patients: A prospective study. *Kidney Int* 1999;**55**:1945–51.

12 Lonnemann G. The quality of dialysate: an integrated approach. *Kidney Int Suppl* 2000;**58**(Suppl 76):S112–19.

13 Lonnemann G. Chronic inflammation in hemodialysis: the role of contaminated dialysate. *Blood Purif* 2000;**18**(3):214–23.

14 Lonnemann G. Should ultra-pure dialysate be mandatory? *Nephrol Dial Transplant* 2000; **15**(Suppl 1):55–9.

15 Ward RA. Ultrapure dialysate: a desirable and achievable goal for routine hemodialysis. *Semin Dial* 2000;**13**(6):378–80.

16 Mion CM, Hegstrom RM, Boen ST *et al*. Substitution of sodium acetate for sodium bicarbonate in the bath fluid for hemodialysis. *Trans Am Soc Artif Intern Organs* 1964; **10**:110–15.

17 Novello A, Kelsch RC, Easterling RE. Acetate intolerance during hemodialysis. *Clin Nephrol* 1976;**5**(1):29–32.

18 Aizawa Y, Ohmori T, Imai K *et al*. Depressant action of acetate upon the human cardiovascular system. *Clin Nephrol* 1977;**8**(5):477–80.

19 MacLeod A, Grant A, Donaldson C *et al*. Effectiveness and efficiency of methods of dialysis therapy for end-stage renal disease: systematic reviews. *Health Technol Assess* 1998;**2**(5):1–166.

20 Veech RL. The untoward effects of the anions of dialysis fluids. *Kidney Int* 1988;**34**:587–97.

21 Jackson MA, Holland MR, Nicholas J *et al*. Occult hypoglycemia caused by hemodialysis. *Clin Nephrol* 1999;**51**(4):242–7.

22 Catalano C, Bordin V, Fabbian F *et al*. Glucose-free standard hemodialysis and occult hypoglycemia. *Clin Nephrol* 2000;**53**(3):235–6.

23 MacLeod A, Daly C, Khan IH *et al*. *Comparison of cellulose, modified cellulose and synthetic membranes in the haemodialysis of patients with end-stage renal disease* (Cochrane Review). Oxford: Update Software, 2001.

24 Foley RN, Parfrey PS, Harnett JD *et al*. Hypoalbuminemia, cardiac morbidity, and mortality in end-stage renal disease. *J Am Soc Nephrol* 1996;**7**(5):728–36.

25 Goldwasser P, Mittman N, Antignani A *et al*. Predictors of mortality in hemodialysis patients. *J Am Soc Nephrol* 1993;**3**:1613–22.

26 Iseki K, Uehara H, Nishime K *et al*. Impact of the initial levels of laboratory variables on survival in chronic dialysis patients. *Am J Kidney Dis* 1996;**28**(4):541–8.

27 Iseki K, Miyasato F, Tokuyama K *et al*. Low diastolic blood pressure, hypoalbuminemia, and risk of death in a cohort of chronic hemodialysis patients. *Kidney Int* 1997;**51**(4):1212–17.

28 Owen WF, Lew NL, Lowrie EG *et al*. The urea reduction ratio and serum albumin concentration as predictors of mortality in patients undergoing hemodialysis. *N Engl J Med* 1993;**329**:1001–06.

29 Greenwood RN. An incremental high-flux dialysis/hemodiafiltration program based on urea kinetic modelling. *Semin Dial* 1999;**12**(Suppl 1):S71–5.

30 Tokars JI, Miller ER, Alter MJ, Arduino MJ. National surveillance of dialysis-associated diseases in the United States, 1997. *Semin Dial* 2000;**13**(2):75–85.

31 Wing AJ, Brunner FP, Brynger HO *et al*. Mortality and morbidity of reusing dialysers. A report by the registration committee of the European Dialysis and Transplant Association. *BMJ* 1978;**2**(6141): 853–5.

32 Pollak VE, Kant KS, Parnell SL *et al*. Repeated use of dialyzers is safe: long-term observations on morbidity and mortality in patients with end-stage renal disease. *Nephron* 1986;**42**(3):217–23.

33 Held PJ, Pauly MV, Diamond L. Survival analysis of patients undergoing dialysis. *JAMA* 1987;**257**(5):645–50.

34 Port FK, Wolfe RA, Hulbert-Shearon TE *et al*. Mortality risk by hemodialyzer reuse practice and dialyzer membrane characteristics: results from the USRDS dialysis morbidity and mortality study. *Am J Kidney Dis* 2001;**37**(2):276–86.

35   Port FK, Orzol SM, Held PJ, Wolfe RA. Trends in treatment and survival for hemodialysis patients in the United States. *Am J Kidney Dis* 1998;**32**(Suppl 4):S34–8.

36   Lowrie EG, Parker TF, Parker TF, Sargent JA. Effect of the hemodialysis prescription of patient morbidity: report from the National Cooperative Dialysis Study. *N Engl J Med* 1981;**305**(20):1176–81.

37   Lowrie EG, Teehan BP. Principles of prescribing dialysis therapy: implementing recommendations from the National Cooperative Dialysis Study. *Kidney Int Suppl* 1983;**13**:S113–22.

38   Goodkin DA, Dickma DM, Rasmussa CS *et al*. Components of hemodialysis dose: results from 7 countries in the Dialysis Outcomes and Practice Patterns Study (DOPPS) (abstract). *J Am Soc Nephrol* 2000;**11**:320A.

39   Mastrangelo F, Alfonso L, Napoli M *et al*. Dialysis with increased frequency of sessions (Lecce dialysis). *Nephrol Dial Transplant* 1998;**13**(Suppl 6):139–47.

40   Raj DS, Charra B, Pierratos A, Work J. In search of ideal hemodialysis: is prolonged frequent dialysis the answer? *Am J Kidney Dis* 1999;**34**(4):597–610.

41   Galland R, Traeger J, Arkouche W *et al*. Short daily hemodialysis and nutritional status. *Am J Kidney Dis* 2001;**37**(Suppl 2):S95–8.

42   Twardowski ZJ. Daily dialysis: is this a reasonable option for the new millennium? *Nephrol Dial Transplant* 2001;**16**(7):1321–4.

43   Deptnor T. Haemodialysis kinetic modelling. In: Henrich WL (ed). *The principles and practice of dialysis*, 2nd edn. Philadelphia: Lippincott, Williams and Wilkins,1999: Chapter 7.

44   Gotch F. Urea kinetic modelling to guide haemodialysis therapy in adults. In: Nissenson AR, Fine RN (eds). *Dialysis therapy*, 2nd edn. Philadelphia: Hanley and Belfus, 2002;Section 6:117–21.

45   Sherman RA, Hootkins R. Simplified formulas for monitoring haemodialysis adequacy. In: Nissenson AR, Fine RN (eds). *Dialysis therapy*, 3rd edn. Philadelphia: Hanley and Belfus, 2002;Section 6:122–6.

46   Lowrie EG, Lew NL. The urea reduction ratio (URR): A simple method for evaluating hemodialysis treatment. *Contemp Dial Nephrol* 1991;**12**(2):11–20.

47   Depner TA. Assessing adequacy of hemodialysis: urea modeling. *Kidney Int* 1994;**45**(5):1522–35.

48   Sherman RA, Cody RP, Rogers ME *et al*. Accuracy of the urea reduction ratio in predicting dialysis delivery. *Kidney Int* 1995;**47**(1):319–21.

49   Parker TF 3rd, Husni L, Huang W *et al*. Survival of hemodialysis patients in the United States is improved with a greater quantity of dialysis. *Am J Kidney Dis* 1994;**23**(5):670–80.

50   Held PJ, Port FK, Wolfe RA *et al*. The dose of hemodialysis and patient mortality. *Kidney Int* 1996;**50**(2):550–6.

51   McClellan WM, Soucie JM, Flanders WD. Mortality in end-stage renal disease is associated with facility-to-facility differences in adequacy of hemodialysis. *J Am Soc Nephrol* 1998;**9**(10):1940–7.

52   Movilli E. Simplified approaches to calculate Kt/V. It's time for agreement. *Nephrol Dial Transplant* 1996;**11**(1):24–7.

53   Gotch FA, Sargent JA. A mechanistic analysis of the National Cooperative Dialysis Study (NCDS). *Kidney Int* 1985;**28**(3):526–34.

54   Held PJ, Levin NW, Bovbjerg RR *et al*. Mortality and duration of hemodialysis treatment. *JAMA* 1991;**265**(7):871–5.

55   Collins AJ, Ma JZ, Umen A *et al*. Urea index and other predictors of hemodialysis patient survival. *Am J Kidney Dis* 1994;**23**(2):272–82.

56   Hakim RM, Breyer J, Ismail N, Schulman G. Effects of dose of dialysis on morbidity and mortality. *Am J Kidney Dis* 1994;**23**(5):661–9.

57   Bloembergen WE, Hakim RM, Stannard DC *et al*. Relationship of dialysis membrane and cause-specific mortality. *Am J Kidney Dis* 1999;**33**(1):1–10.

58   Hornberger JC. The hemodialysis prescription and quality-adjusted life expectancy. Renal Physicians Association Working Committee on Clinical Guidelines. *J Am Soc Nephrol* 1993;**4**(4):1004–20.

59   Hornberger JC. The hemodialysis prescription and cost effectiveness. Renal Physicians Association Working Committee on Clinical Guidelines. *J Am Soc Nephrol* 1993;**4**(4):1021–7.

60   Kjellstrand CM. Duration and adequacy of dialysis. Overview: the science is easy, the ethic is difficult. *ASAIO J* 1997;**43**(3):220–4.

61   Wolfe RA, Ashby VB, Daugirdas JT *et al*. Body size, dose of hemodialysis, and mortality. *Am J Kidney Dis* 2000;**35**(1):80–8.

62   Eknoyan G, Levey AS, Beck GJ *et al*. The hemodialysis (HEMO) study: rationale for selection of interventions. *Semin Dial* 1996;**9**(1):24–33.

63   Lai YH, Guh JY, Chen HC, Tsai JH. Effects of different sampling methods for measurement of post dialysis blood urea nitrogen on urea kinetic modeling derived parameters in patients undergoing long-term hemodialysis. *ASAIO J* 1995;**41**(2):211–15.

64   Tattersall JE, De Takats D, Chammey P *et al*. The post-hemodialysis rebound: predicting and quantifying its effect on Kt/V. *Kidney Int* 1996;**50**(6):2094–102.

65   Tattersall JE, Chammey P, Aldridge C *et al*. Recirculation and the post-dialysis rebound. *Nephrol Dial Transplant* 1996;**11**(Suppl 2):75–80.

66   Daugirdas JT, Smye SW. Effect of a two compartment distribution on apparent urea distribution volume. *Kidney Int* 1997;**51**(4):1270–3.

67   Smye SW, Tattersall JE, Will EJ. Modeling the postdialysis rebound: the reconciliation of current formulas. *ASAIO J* 1999;**45**(6):562–7.

68   Beto JA, Bansal NK, Ing TS *et al*. Variation in blood sample collection for determination of hemodialysis adequacy. Council on Renal Nutrition National Research Question Collaborative Study Group. *Am J Kidney Dis* 1998;**31**(1):135–41.

69   Szczech LA, Lowrie EG, Li Z *et al*. Changing hemodialysis thresholds for optimal survival. *Kidney Int* 2001;**59**(2):738–45.

70   Geddes CC, Traynor J, Walbaum D *et al*. A new method of post-dialysis blood urea sampling: the 'stop dialysate flow' method. *Nephrol Dial Transplant* 2000;**15**(4):517–23.

71   Traynor JP, Geddes CC, Ferguson C, Mactier RA. Predicting 30-minute post-dialysis blood urea concentrations using the stop dialysate flow method. *Am J Kidney Dis* (in press).

72   Ronco C, Brendolan A, Milan M *et al*. Impact of biofeedback-induced cardiovascular stability on hemodialysis tolerance and efficiency. *Kidney Int* 2000;**58**(2):800–8.

73   Daugirdas JT. Dialysis hypotension: a hemodynamic analysis. *Kidney Int* 1991;**39**:233–46.

74   Koch M, Thomas B, Tschope W *et al*. Survival and predictors of death in dialysed diabetic patients. *Diabetologia* 1993;**36**(10):1113–7.

75   Poldermans D, Man in 't Veld AJ, Rambaldi R. Cardiac evaluation in hypotension-prone and hypotension-resistant hemodialysis patients. *Kidney Int* 1999;**56**(5):1905–11.

76   Dheenan S, Henrich WL. Preventing dialysis hypotension: A comparison of usual protective maneuvers. *Kidney Int* 2001;**59**(3):1175–81.

77   Chesser AM, Baker LR. Temporary vascular access for first dialysis is common, undesirable and usually avoidable. *Clin Nephrol* 1999;**51**(4):228–32.

78   Schwab SJ, Beathard G. The hemodialysis catheter conundrum: hate living with them, but can't live without them. *Kidney Int* 1999;**56**(1):1–17.

79   Schwab SJ, Harrington JT, Singh A *et al*. Vascular access for hemodialysis. *Kidney Int* 1999;**55**(5):2078–90.

80   Nassar GM, Ayus JC. Infectious complications of hemodialysis access. *Kidney Int* 2001;**60**(1):1–13.

81   Pisoni RL, Young EW, Dykstra DM *et al*. Vascular access use in Europe and the United States; Results from the DOPPS. *Kidney Int* 2002;**61**:305–16.

82   Ansell D, Feest T (eds). The UK Renal Registry. *The second annual report*, 1999. Bristol: UK Renal Registry, 1999;175–87.

83 Warady BA, Sullivan EK, Alexander SR. Lessons from the patient database. *Kidney Int* 1996;**49**:S68–71.

84 Alexander SR, Harmon WE, Jabs K. Dialysis in Children. In: Henrich WL (ed). *Principles and practice of dialysis*. Baltimore MD: Williams and Wilkins, 1994;404.

85 Furth SL, Powe NR, Hwang W. Does greater paediatric experience influence treatment choice in chronic disease management? *Arch Pediatr Adolescent Med* 1997;**151**:545–50.

86 Royal College of Nursing. *Paediatric nephrology nursing. Guidance for nurses*. London: RCN, November 2000.

87 Wilson L. The home visiting programme. *Paediatr Nursing* 1995; July 10–11.

88 Sharma A, Zillerueb G, Abitbol C *et al*. Survival and complications of cuffed catheters in children on haemodialysis. *Pediatr Nephrol* 1999;**13**:245–8.

89 Smoyer W, Sherbotie J, Gardner J, Bunchman T. A practical approach to continuous haemofiltration in infants and children. *Dial and Transplant* 1995;**24**(11):663–40.

90 Hoenich NA, Woffindin G, Ronco C. Haemodialysis and associate devices. In: Jacobs C, Kjellstrand CM, Koch KM, Winchester JF (eds). *Replacement of renal function by dialysis*, 4th edn. Dordrecht: Kluwer Academic Publishers, 1996:188.

91 Goldstein SL, Sorof JM, Brewer ED. Natural logarithmic estimates of Kt/V in the pediatric dialysis population. *Am J Kidney Dis* 1999;**33**:518–22.

92 Watson AR, Gartland C. Avoiding and coping with patient and family burnout. In: Fine RN, Alexander SR, Warady BA (eds). *CAPD/CCPD in children*, 2nd edn. Boston: Kluwer Academic Publishers 1998;491–506.

93 Beadles E, Stephenson R, Watson AR. Kidney failure at school. *Family Medicine* 1997;**1**:11–13.

94 Watson AR, Shooter M. Transitioning adolescents from paediatric to adult dialysis units. In: Khanna R (ed). *Advances in peritoneal dialysis*. Toronto: Peritoneal Dialysis Publications Inc, 1996;176–8.

95 Challah S, Wing AJ, Bauer R *et al*. Negative selection of patients for dialysis in the United Kingdom. *Br Med J* 1984;**288**:1119–22.

96 Hirsch DJ, West ML, Cohen AD, Jindal KK. Experience with not offering dialysis to patients with a poor prognosis. *Am J Kidney Dis* 1994;**23**:463–6.

97 Main J. Deciding not to start dialysis – a one year prospective study in Teesside. *J Nephrol* 1000;**13**:137–41.

98 Catalano C, Goodship THJ, Graham KA *et al*. Withdrawal of renal replacement therapy in Newcastle upon Tyne: 1964-1993. *Nephrol Dial Transplant* 1996;**11**:133–9.

99 Cohen LM, McCue JD, Germain M, Kjellstrand CJ. Dialysis discontinued: a "good" death? *Arch Intern Med* 1995;**155**:42–7.

100 Friedman EA. The best and worst times for dialysis are now. *ASAIO J* 1994;**40**:107–08.

101 Singer J, Thiel EC, Naylor D *et al*. Life-sustaining treatment preferences of hemodialysis patients: implications for advance directives. *J Am Soc Nephrol* 1995;**6**:1410–17.

102 Tobe SW, Senn JS (for the End-Stage Renal Disease Group). Foregoing renal dialysis: case study and review of ethical issues. *Am J Kidney Dis* 1996;**28**:147–53.

103 Campbell ML. Terminal care of ESRD patients forgoing dialysis. *ANNA J* 1991;**18**:202–04.

104 Cohen LM, Germian M, Poppel DM *et al*. Dialysis discontinuation and palliative care. *Am J Kidney Dis* 2000;140–4.

105 Association for the Advancement of Medical Instrumentation. Draft Standard RD 62-D: Water treatment equipment for hemodialysis applications. Arlington, VA: AAMI, 2001.

4 | Peritoneal dialysis

Introduction

4.1   Peritoneal dialysis (PD) is a well-established treatment modality for end stage renal disease (ESRD), providing both patients and clinicians with additional choice and flexibility. On average, it is the initial treatment for 30–40% of patients in the UK, although local practice does vary.

Equipment and fluids*

Standards

▶ A unit offering PD should provide not only continuous ambulatory peritoneal dialysis (CAPD) but also automated peritoneal dialysis (APD), in all its forms. It should have access to adequate back-up haemodialysis (HD) facilities and renal transplantation. **(Good practice)**

▶ All equipment used in the delivery and monitoring of therapies should comply with the relevant standards for medical electrical equipment (BS-EN 50072:1992, BS 5724-2.29:1992, IEC 60601–2–39:1998. Medical electrical equipment. Particular requirements for safety. Specification for peritoneal dialysis equipment). Tubing sets and catheters should carry the CE mark to indicate that the item conforms to the essential requirements of the Medical Devices Directive (93/42/EEC) and that its conformity has been assessed in accordance with the Directive. **(Good practice)**

▶ Fluids for PD are required to satisfy the current European quality standards as indicated in the European good manufacturing practice and the European Pharmacopoeia Monograph, *Solutions for peritoneal dialysis*. Manufacturing facilities are required to meet the relevant standards (ISO 9001/2 and EN 46001/2). Product registration files must be submitted to, and product approval given by, the Medicines Control Agency. **(Good practice)**

▶ The use of disconnect systems should be standard unless clinically contraindicated. **(A)**

Recommendations

▶ The unit should be aware of the limitations of CAPD and related techniques. **(B)**

▶ In selected patients – those with high small solute transfer rates and little or no residual function – specialised solutions such as glucose polymers (icodextrin) are preferable to standard solutions. **(B)**

▶ APD should be available as clinically indicated and not constrained by financial considerations. **(C)**

*See Appendix D for details of standards abbreviations used in this section.

RATIONALE

4.2   Disconnect 'flush before fill' systems are superior to earlier systems. In controlled trials, their use results in a significantly lower incidence of peritonitis and a better quality of life.[1,2] In a recent systematic review, peritonitis occurred significantly less frequently using the Y-set/modified Y-set compared with the standard spike system. The former was also more cost-efficient if it is assumed that there is a higher technique failure rate with the spike or non-disconnect systems.[3] Such systems should be standard for all patients, unless they are incapable of managing this slightly more difficult technique. Extra costs should be partly offset by lower morbidity, hospital admission and peritoneal failure rates.[4]

4.3   In patients with large muscle mass and no or little residual renal function, it may be difficult to provide adequate dialysis.[5] The survival of PD patients is at least as good as those on HD over the first 2–4 years.[6] Positive reasons for opting for PD include preservation of residual renal function and vascular access sites, reduced delayed graft function following transplantation and increased patient autonomy. The last is of particular importance to patients who wish to travel or remain in employment, or to those caring for children/relatives, and is often further facilitated by the use of APD.

4.4   The use of cycling machines at home may be necessary for clinical reasons, for example, high transporter status of the peritoneum (10–15% of the dialysis population), or impaired filtration, or for psychosocial reasons; these three groups form 20–25% of the total CAPD population. In addition, patient preference should be considered when prescribing APD. As yet, there have been no studies on the long-term outcome of patients treated by APD as a first option, in comparison with CAPD. Monitoring of the dose of dialysis delivered is especially important in APD (see below and Appendix 1). Automated systems are more expensive than standard disconnect manual systems; their extra costs will need to be reflected in contracts negotiated with purchasers, but it should be noted that usually APD will be cheaper for such patients than the alternative, ie transfer to in-centre HD.

4.5   Icodextrin may have particular value in improving ultrafiltration in patients with high small-solute transfer rates and little or no residual function. It has been claimed that use of this fluid will extend time on PD.[7,8] Thus, the increased cost of icodextrin may be more than offset by the saving in total modality cost achieved by avoiding a transfer to HD. Other solutions with variations in the concentration of sodium, calcium, magnesium, osmotic agents and buffers (bicarbonate) may also be required. Such solutions are likely to be more expensive, so their selective use should be reflected in negotiations with commissioners.

Testing membrane function and dialysis adequacy   4.6   Observational studies have shown that solute clearance and membrane function are independent predictors of patient and technique survival, at least in CAPD patients. Hence, the following recommendations emphasise the need to measure membrane function and solute clearance, and give minimum targets for the latter. The relationship mentioned above between clinical outcome and solute clearance is, however, essentially due to the influence of residual renal function, and it is increasingly clear that residual renal and peritoneal clearances cannot be considered as equivalent.

▶ A peritoneal equilibration test (PET) should be performed after 4–8 weeks on dialysis, and when clinically indicated, eg when biochemical indices or loss of ultrafiltration raise suspicion of changes in peritoneal transport characteristics, or when therapy is changed to APD. **(C)**

▶ A total weekly creatinine clearance (dialysis + residual renal function) of greater than 50 l/week/1.73 m^2 and/or a weekly dialysis Kt/V urea of greater than 1.7, checked eight weeks after beginning dialysis, are minima. Higher targets are desirable especially for high average and high transporters and APD patients. **(B)**

▶ At present both Kt/V and creatinine clearance are acceptable measures of adequacy until evidence accumulates to show the superiority of one over the other. Achieving either target is acceptable; creatinine clearance is more difficult to achieve in anuric patients with below average peritoneal solute transport. **(C)**

▶ These studies should be repeated at least annually, and more frequently if clinically indicated, particularly if suspicion arises that residual renal function has declined more rapidly than usual. **(C)**

▶ Careful attention to fluid balance, especially in anuric patients, is essential. The use of icodextrin in the day-time dwell combined with APD to achieve both adequate solute clearances and fluid removal is recommended. **(B)**

RATIONALE

4.7 A peritoneal equilibration test (PET)[9] is used to assess peritoneal membrane function, in particular loss of ultrafiltration.[10] It measures the peritoneal membrane transporter status and the ultrafiltration capacity. It is essential in prescribing the appropriate PD regimen, but is not a measure of treatment adequacy. Membrane function takes 4–6 weeks after starting dialysis to stabilise.[11] Inadequate ultrafiltration should be suspected in patients with high solute transport or an ultrafiltration capacity <200 ml.[12] The standard permeability analysis (SPA), which uses a 3.86% glucose dwell (as opposed to the PET which uses 2.27%) over four hours, defines ultrafiltration failure as <400 ml ultrafiltration capacity, in the absence of fluid leak or catheter malfunction.[13] The additional measurement of the sodium dialysate/plasma (D/P) ratio at one hour gives an estimation of sodium sieving across the peritoneal vasculature, which if absent indicates poor ultrafiltration.

4.8 After 4–8 weeks, a PET should be done to assess peritoneal transport characteristics. Patients with high transport characteristics may not be suitable for standard CAPD exchanges, and will often require short-dwell APD. There is now good evidence that the outcome (patient and technique survival) is worse in high transporters.[14–16] In these patients greater emphasis on fluid control may be necessary.[17] Those with low transporter status may be unsuitable for APD altogether, unless they have good residual renal function (see 4.13 and 4.15). However, it has been demonstrated that patients with low transport have good outcomes on CAPD, probably because they ultrafiltrate well and are less likely to have fluid overload.

4.9 It is believed that the concept of adequacy, including the dose of dialysis, is very important. It has been shown in prospective studies to be a predictor of outcome in new patients starting CAPD[18–20] and in patients already on CAPD treatment.[21,22] As with patients on HD, adequacy is a global concept, involving various levels of measurement, which include clinical assessment of well-being and physical measurements, measures of small molecule solute clearance and fluid removal, and the impact of the treatment on the patient's life. It is important that clinical aspects be taken into consideration in arriving at targets of small molecule solute clearance, which in general are the basis for measuring dialysis dose.

4.10   Prospective cohort studies in which peritoneal dialysis dose was unadjusted[18–20] have reported reduced survival in patients in whom creatinine and urea clearances were not maintained. In these studies, the influence of clearances on survival could be attributed almost entirely to the maintenance of residual renal function. These studies also identified an independent increased risk of patient death and technical failure as peritoneal solute transport increased. This observation is likely to be explained by impaired fluid balance in CAPD patients with higher solute transport. The implications of these findings are that PD patients who have lost residual renal function are at increased risk, due to a combination of reduced clearance and fluid removal.

4.11   There is some evidence that CAPD patients are chronically fluid overloaded,[17] and this impacts on cardiovascular outcomes.[23] In addition, patients who have no residual renal function (Canada and USA Collaboration Study (CANUSA)) or those with high peritoneal solute transport have a less favourable outcome.[24] This may in part reflect poor fluid control, increased hypertension and left ventricular hypertrophy (LVH).[25] There is no simple, direct way of assessing fluid status in PD patients, but studies of body composition suggest that greater attention to fluid balance is necessary. Loss of ultrafiltration is not uncommon in long-term PD patients.[19] Recently, management guidelines by the International Society for Peritoneal Dialysis (ISPD) have been published[26] which outline the approach to managing a PD patient with fluid overload. Particular care should be taken in anuric patients treated with APD, due to the risk of fluid re-absorption during the day-time dwell. A randomised study of APD patients, comparing day-time ultrafiltration with 2.27% glucose verses icodextrin, found that the latter achieved better fluid removal.[27] A recent, uncontrolled study demonstrated improvement in body fluid composition in APD patients switched to icodextrin during the day-time dwell.[28]

4.12   Prescribing of dialysis dose and measurement of adequacy of dialysis are best done during the initiation phase immediately after starting CAPD, and in a subsequent phase when the dose is assessed and monitored. Since the PET takes 4–6 weeks to stabilise (see 4.7), values obtained earlier than this may not be representative of membrane transport characteristics in the longer term. Hence the initial CAPD regimen should be prescribed assuming normal transport characteristics, the measured residual renal function (RRF) and body surface area. Subsequently, in the light of PET results, the definitive prescription is arrived at, and is adjusted to meet targets of solute clearance (see 4.14) and fluid removal according to fluctuations in dwell times, fill volumes, glucose concentration and change to APD.

4.13   The weekly Kt/V for urea and the weekly creatinine clearance are both used at present as measures of small solute clearance. Each is the sum of the clearance achieved by the dialysis and that due to the RRF. Renal and peritoneal clearance are not equal, although this is assumed when compensating for the loss of RRF by increasing peritoneal clearances. At present, the two measures (Kt/V and creatinine clearance) are regarded as being equivalent and either can be used. Creatinine clearance is greatly affected by RRF and declines more as RRF decreases. Also, these two measurements differ in their susceptibility to manipulation; in practice, creatinine clearance is much more difficult to increase than Kt/V for urea; the National Kidney Foundation Dialysis Outcome Quality Initiative (DOQI) guidelines in the USA have given preference to Kt/V measurements.[29]

4.14   A weekly Kt/V <1.65 was reported to be associated with poor outcomes.[30,31] A weekly Kt/V >2.0 (dialysis + RRF) or total weekly creatinine clearance of >60 l/week/1.73 m^2 of body surface area has been advocated for standard CAPD.[29] The Canadian guidelines recommend a minimum target Kt/V of 2.0 but a creatinine clearance of 60 l/week/1.73 m^2 for high and high average transporters, and 50 l/week/1.73 m^2 for low and low average transporters.[32] Higher clearances have been suggested.[33,34] It must be emphasised also that all these studies were based largely on theoretical predictions, even though these have been validated to some extent against actual experience,[35] and that there is no final proof that achieving these targets will result in improved outcome.[36] The recently reported Mexican Adequacy randomised control trial (ADEMEX)[37] showed no difference in outcome after two years in patients maintaining a creatinine clearance of 46 litres per week compared with those achieving 57 litres per week. This study therefore provides a firmer evidence base and justifies the minimum target of creatinine clearance of 50 litres per week and a Kt/V greater than 1.7. In the CANUSA study,[18] three-quarters of the deaths during treatment within two years of starting CAPD were from cardiovascular causes, some in well dialysed patients. Solute clearance also affects morbidity (hospitalisations, peritonitis), although the level of solute clearance where this becomes relevant is uncertain. The link between adequacy and nutrition is present, but hitherto has been based on cross-sectional data of a significant correlation between Kt/V and protein catabolic rate (PCR), which is a mathematical artifact of the use of V to calculate both parameters;[38] it should not be used to assess the impact of adequacy of dialysis on nutrition. There is evidence that increasing the delivered dialysis dose is feasible, and has modest beneficial effects in malnourished patients, without co-morbidity,[39] and in reducing hospitalisation rates.[40]

4.15   As mentioned in the introduction to this chapter, APD comprises a number of regimes involving varying amounts of fluid and dwell times. These include continuous cycler assisted PD (CCPD), nocturnal intermittent PD (NIPD), NIPD with 'wet' days (dialysis done during the day), and tidal PD. There are few data on either solute clearances or impact on outcome of such regimes. With the current recommendation for solute clearance,[29] it seems that a 'wet day' is going to be necessary to augment clearances. At present, there is no evidence to support the higher targets of solute clearance advocated for APD regimes, most of which are continuous therapies.

4.16   Thus, the recommendations given immediately above can be regarded as approximate targets for which to aim, and can be refined in the light of future data. Again we emphasise that the general condition of the patient must be taken into account when prescribing the quantity of CAPD; a well nourished patient with good biochemistry and haemoglobin but apparently unsatisfactory clearance is preferable to an ill patient with poor metabolic control but apparently good clearance.

4.17　As emphasised above, decline in RRF has an important bearing on the adequacy of dialysis. Consequently, RRF should be assessed at least annually as part of the assessment of total adequacy, or whenever under-dialysis is suspected.[41] Measurement of RRF is described in Appendix 1. There is evidence that the regular use of a loop diuretic can maintain urine volume for longer, without affecting clearances, although whether this will affect outcome is unknown.[42] A loop diuretic may be prescribed, if there is no contraindication, to all PD patients.

Infective complications

4.18　Infection continues to be the most important complication of PD. This is especially the case for peritonitis, which still causes between 30% and 50% of technical failures.

Recommendations

▶ Peritonitis rates should be <1 episode/18 patient months. **(A)**

▶ The negative peritoneal fluid culture rate in patients with clinical peritonitis should be less than 15%. **(B)**

▶ The initial cure rate of peritonitis should be more than 80% (without necessitating catheter removal). **(B)**

▶ Mupirocin should be used as part of routine exit-site care; daily or on alternate days. **(B)**

▶ Nasal application of mupirocin in *Staphylococcus aureus* carriers should be undertaken twice daily for five consecutive days every four weeks. **(A)**

RATIONALE

4.19　Peritonitis is the major and most serious complication of CAPD. Apart from the immediate deleterious effects and distress of the acute episode, there is mounting evidence that repeated attacks of peritonitis are associated with earlier failure of the peritoneal membrane. How the frequency of episodes of peritonitis should be measured and expressed remains a subject of controversy. In some studies, episodes within a short and variable period of either catheter insertion or beginning dialysis are excluded, and in other studies included. In general an actuarial analysis of time free of peritonitis is the best way to express the peritonitis rate,[1,43] and we advocate its use, but this has been little used in clinical practice. Despite its theoretical and practical disadvantages, the number of episodes/unit time remains in widest use, and the recommendation is couched in these terms.

4.20　Peritonitis rates are improving with the introduction of disconnect systems.[7] The successful diagnosis and management of peritonitis requires high quality microbiological facilities and close liaison with the microbiology department. Protocols for managing peritonitis episodes have been published.[44,45] It must be noted that the use of vancomycin as a first-line 'blind' antibiotic has been curtailed recently because of the emergence of vancomycin-resistant organisms,[46] and alternative regimens have not been evaluated so extensively.[47] With the occurrence of more unusual organisms causing peritonitis the initial cure rate may fall.

4.21   Guidelines for the insertion of peritoneal access catheters and their subsequent care have been published[48] and we advocate the use of these. The essential guidelines from this report are:

1   Overall no catheter appears to be superior to the standard double cuff Tenckhoff catheter.

2   A downward directed exit site decreases the incidence of catheter-related infections.

3   The insertion must be done by a competent and experienced operator.

Other recommendations relate to details of post-operative care, management of catheter-related infections and non-infectious (mechanical) catheter-related complications.

4.22   Catheter-related infections (exit-site, tunnel) with subsequent peritonitis account for up to 20% of transfers to HD.[49] Their prevention is important. Nasal carriage of *Staphylococcus aureus* (the most common organism causing catheter infections) is now strongly linked with exit-site infections.[50] Antibiotic prophylaxis (application of mupirocin ointment to the exit-site) in carriers has shown up to 50% reduction in catheter-related infections and, in these patients, is of clear value.[51] Regular screening for nasal *S. aureus* carriage is time consuming, however, and an alternative strategy of using mupirocin as part of the routine exit-site care in all patients has been advocated. A recent sequential prospective study using this approach has shown a dramatic reduction in exit-site infections and peritonitis when compared to historical controls.[52] This approach is advocated, but clinicians will need to work with their local microbiologists to implement it, and caution needs to be exercised with respect to development of resistance to mupirocin; this has not been shown to occur in 12 months of prophylactic use at the exit-site.[53] Studies to date have followed patients for up to 18 months. It is not yet clear whether several years usage of mupirocin is necessary or desirable.

Paediatric section

Equipment, fluids and personnel

Standard

▶ All children requiring PD should be treated in a designated paediatric nephrology and dialysis centre. (**Good practice**)

Recommendations

▶ It is essential that the child and family are prepared for PD by a renally trained children's nurse with appropriate written information. Preparation by the nurse and/or play specialist will also include aids such as dolls or videos.[54] (**Good practice**)

▶ Problems with needle phobia will require referral to a child psychologist. (**Good practice**)

▶ Insertion of the chronic peritoneal catheter should be by an appropriately trained surgeon. (**Good practice**)

▶ Training in the management of PD should be supervised by a paediatric renal nurse. (**Good practice**)

▶ The child's nutritional status needs to be managed and monitored by a paediatric renal dietitian.[55] (**Good practice**)

▶ Since the home environment and the impact on the family are so important for the success of PD, psychosocial support such as liaison visits to the home, nursery or school and GP should be provided by the dialysis nurse and other team members such as social workers.[54] (**Good practice**)

RATIONALE

4.23   The greater use of PD has enabled infants with ESRD to be treated from birth when appropriate. These infants require additional intensive medical and nutritional support and their associated urological abnormalities emphasise the need for management in paediatric nephrology and dialysis centres.[56] Families should be actively involved in the choice of therapy, taking into account the difficulties of vascular access in small children, large distances from the paediatric dialysis centre, co-morbidity factors and the level of family support available.

4.24   There is increasing awareness of the unfavourable properties of glucose as an osmotic agent. Since the preferred treatment modality in children is APD, dwell times are usually short. This makes the application of a pH neutral dialysis solution for the standard nightly prescription highly desirable, but such solutions still need to be evaluated. If ultrafiltration is insufficient using the standard regimen, then the addition of a long daytime dwell with polyglucose solutions should be considered. Long-term studies of this subject in paediatrics are lacking. The place of amino acid-containing dialysis fluid still has to be determined in paediatric PD.[57]

4.25   Continuous peritoneal dialysis (CPD) is the favoured dialysis modality in children of all ages in the UK, with 79 children under 15 years of age on PD compared with 56 on HD in the UK in 2000.[58] Overnight APD is the commonest and most appropriate form of PD for young children. This is because the predominantly fluid diet means that the dialysis must remove large volumes of fluid, which is best achieved during the long hours that a young child spends asleep. APD has also been advocated for children as this gives greater freedom during the day for school and social activities, which are an important part of their development.

Testing membrane function and dialysis adequacy

Recommendations

▶ A PET and measurement of adequacy parameters should be undertaken annually but should be considered sooner if there is growth failure. (**Good practice**)

▶ Standards of adequacy recommended for adult patients should be regarded as the minimum for children.[59] (**Good practice**)

RATIONALE

4.26   PD adequacy targets have been recommended in adults because patient mortality and morbidity have been much easier to define. There are few data to correlate clinical outcomes with delivered dialysis dose in children because of the smaller number of paediatric patients with varying body size and physical status who often spend shorter periods of time on dialysis before transplantation.

4.27 The efficiency of CPD is to a large part dependent upon the transference properties of the peritoneal membrane. The area of the peritoneal membrane is two-fold larger in infants than in adults at 533 cm^2/kg body weight compared with 284 cm^2/kg body weight respectively, although the surface area is age independent, if expressed per m^2 body surface area (BSA).[60] Therefore scaling of the dialysate fill volume by BSA has been proposed in children to avoid false perception of peritoneal hyperpermeability (as defined in the PET) compared with adults when prescribing fill volumes scaled simply to weight.[61] Exchange volumes should be 1,100–1,400 ml/m^2 BSA, taking into account the tolerance of the volume, the age of the patient, the modality of PD used, ie CAPD or APD, and the time spent on PD.[62]

4.28 A PET is of clinical use in choosing the most appropriate PD modality and guiding the prescription in the individual patient. As in adults, the PET in children should be delayed at least one month from catheter implantation or after a peritonitis episode, and should be performed if membrane failure is suspected or if there is poor growth. There is no firm recommendation for frequency of testing in children but twice per year has been suggested in order to optimise growth.[62]

4.29 Studies in adult patients on PD have characterised dialysis adequacy in terms of small solute clearance and have been based on clinical evidence provided by prospective studies. There are no comparable data available for patients treated by APD. It has been recommended that the delivered dose of nocturnal intermittent peritoneal dialysis (NIPD) should be 8% higher than that of CAPD and that of CCPD should be intermediate between CAPD and NIPD.[63] The few data that are available suggest better growth with better dialysis adequacy.[64] It has been suggested that the recommendations for adults should be regarded as the lower limit of PD prescriptions in children. However, adult adequacy targets should be regarded only as tentative guidelines for children at present; assessment of growth may provide further useful information of dialysis adequacy. Difficulties of 24-hour urine collections in young children make assessment of residual renal function inaccurate. The benefits of increasing PD doses have to be balanced against the cost in terms of the child's social rehabilitation and quality of life.

Infective complications

Standard

▶ A minimum peritonitis rate of <1 episode per 14 patient months is recommended, averaged over three years. (**Good practice**)

RATIONALE

4.30 Peritonitis rates show a great variation between units on an annual audit because of the small number of patients in any one centre and the distorting effect of some patients, eg infants. Gastrostomies, vesicostomies and ureterostomies are not contra-indications to CPD in children. Peritonitis rates in children have improved in recent years with rates in Europe currently being <1 episode in 20 patient months,[65] although a recent German multicentre trial reported a rate of one episode per 13.7 patient months.[66] We await definitive British data but a minimum standard of <1 episode per 14 patient months is recommended, averaged over three years.

4.31 There is no firm agreement on the best catheter configuration to use in children, as there are no conclusive data on the impact on peritonitis rates. However, different sizes of catheter are required in children of different body weights.[54,67] Data from the North American Registry suggest that children should have PD catheters that have swan neck tunnels, two cuffs and downward pointing exit sites.[68] All catheter connections should be luerlock. Although there are no specific paediatric studies, disconnect 'flush before fill' systems such as Y-sets should be routine for CAPD. There are no conclusive studies on the standard care of the PD catheter exit site in children. In general, adult recommendations are followed.[67] After a successful renal transplant, rejection episodes requiring a return to dialysis are rare after the first month, but catheter-related infections increase at this time.[69] The recommended time for removal of the PD catheter is therefore 3–6 weeks following successful transplantation.

Psycho-social support

See the standards and recommendations on p.32, Chapter 3.

Research and audit

Recommendation

▶ Each paediatric renal unit should maintain mortality and morbidity data for patients on CPD. All PD-related problems, such as catheter malfunction rates, exit-site and tunnel infections and peritonitis rates, and results of dialysis adequacy parameters and their relationship to growth, should be maintained by each unit. The data should be submitted to the British Paediatric Renal Registry. (**Good epidemiological practice**)

Appendix 1: Methods for assessment of membrane function and solute clearance in peritoneal dialysis

Assessment of membrane function

A number of methods to assess the peritoneal membrane have been developed, the most commonly used being the peritoneal equilibration test (PET), supported by clinical observation. This test measures two aspects of membrane function: low molecular weight solute transport (expressed as the dialysate:plasma ratio of creatinine at four hours), and the ultrafiltration capacity of the membrane. In the PET as originally described, ultrafiltration capacity is the net volume of ultrafiltration achieved at four hours using a 2.27% glucose exchange.[9] In the simplified standard permeability analysis (SPA) test, it is the net volume of ultrafiltration using a 3.86% exchange.[13]

The clinical value of assessing membrane function is as follows:

▶ Solute transport rates vary considerably in the PD population and inform dialysis prescription, allowing optimisation of both solute clearance and ultrafiltration.

▶ In CAPD patients, high solute transport is associated with reduced technical and patients survival. These patients may benefit from APD and polyglucose solutions.[15,16] Solute transport can change with time on treatment, and is the most common cause of ultrafiltration failure.[54] Using a standard PET, an ultrafiltration capacity of <200 ml is associated with a 50% risk of achieving <1,000 ml ultrafiltration in anuric patients.[55] Using an SPA test, an ultrafiltration capacity of <400 ml indicates ultrafiltration failure.[13]

The methods of performing PET and SPA tests are well described in the literature. The following points should be remembered in the interpretation of results:

▶ High concentrations of glucose interfere with many assays for creatinine. It is important to work with the local biochemists to ensure that the appropriate correction for measurement of creatinine in dialysate has been taken into account. The patient should follow their usual dialysate regimen, draining out as completely as possible before the test dwell. Large residual volume of dialysate will affect the results. Intra-patient variability of the ultrafiltration capacity (~20%) is greater than for the solute transport (<10%). Results of the PET/SPA, in particular the ultrafiltration capacity, should always be interpreted in the light of additional exchanges performed during the same 24–48 hour period (usually collected to assess solute clearance – see below). The PET/SPA tests are not surrogates for measuring solute clearance.

Measurement of solute clearance

In measuring solute clearance and planning changes to the dialysis regimen, three clinical parameters are essential. These are estimates of:

1   Patient size

2   Peritoneal solute transport

3   RRF.

In each case, the choice of surrogate 'toxin', urea or creatinine, interacts with each of these parameters in different ways. At present, there is no clear evidence from the literature that one surrogate is superior to another. Where possible, clinicians should measure both, attempt to reach at least one of the targets, and understand why there appears to be a discrepancy. A number of commercial computer programs exist that are designed to aid dialysis prescription. Whilst some have been validated, good practice dictates that a change in dialysis prescription is checked for efficacy by repeating clearance studies.

Patient size

In calculating urea clearances, patient size is expressed as an estimate of the total body water (volume of distribution of urea). It is recommended that the Watson formula is used for this:

Males: $V = 2.447 - 0.09156 \times \text{age (years)} + 0.1074 \times \text{height (cm)} + 0.3362 \times \text{weight (kg)}$

Females: $V = -2.097 + 0.1069 \times \text{age (years)} + 0.2466 \times \text{weight (kg)}$

Alternatively 58% of body weight (kg) may be used; this is less precise, and will give lower values for Kt/V, especially in obese patients. Creatinine clearances should be corrected for body surface area, normalising to 1.73 m^2.

Peritoneal solute transport

Solute transport rates have an important influence on peritoneal creatinine clearance, but not on urea clearance. This means that it is easier to achieve creatinine clearance targets in high transport patients. It should be remembered, however, that these patients might have less satisfactory ultrafiltration. In designing optimum dialysis regimens, patients with low solute transport will require equally spaced medium length dwells, such as are achieved with CAPD and single extra night exchanges (eg 5 × 2.5 litre exchanges). Those with high transport are more likely to achieve targets with short dwells (APD) plus polyglucose solutions (eg 4 × 2.5 litre exchanges overnight, 1 × 2.5 litre evening exchange and 1 × 2.5 litre daytime icodextrin).

Residual renal function (RRF)

This is the single most important parameter in PD patients, and also the one most likely to change with time. Clinically significant changes can occur within three months. Because secretion of creatinine by the kidney at low levels of function over-estimates residual creatinine clearance, it is recommended that this should be expressed as the mean of the urea and creatinine clearances.

References

1   Maiorca R, Cantaluppi A, Cancarini GC *et al.* Prospective controlled trial of a Y-connector and disinfectant to prevent peritonitis in continuous ambulatory peritoneal dialysis. *Lancet* 1983;2: 642–4.

2   Churchill DN, Taylor DW, Vas SL. Peritonitis in CAPD: a multicentre randomised clinincal trial comparing the Y connector disinfectant system to standard systems. *Perit Dial Int* 1989;9:159–63.

3   Daly C, Campbell M, Cody J *et al.* Double bag or Y-set versus standard transfer systems for continuous ambulatory peritoneal dialysis in end stage renal disease. Cochrane Renal Group. Cochrane Database of Systematic Reviews. Issue 2, 2001.

4   Harris DC, Yuill EJ, Byth K *et al.* Twin- versus single-bag disconnect systems: infection rates and cost of continuous ambulatory peritoneal dialysis. *J Am Soc Nephrol* 1996;7:2392–8.

5   Tzamaloukas AH, Murata GH, Malhotra D *et al.* Creatinine clearance in continuous peritoneal dialysis: dialysis dose required for a minimal acceptable level. *Perit Dial Int* 1996;16:41–7.

6   Fenton SSA, Schaubel DE, Desmeules M *et al.* Hemodialysis versus peritoneal dialysis: a comparison of adjusted mortality rates. *Am J Kidney Dis* 1997;30:334–42.

7   Mistry CD, Gokal R. Icodextrin in peritoneal dialysis: early development and clinical use. *Perit Dial Int* 1994;14:S13–21.

8   Wilkie M, Plant MJ, Edwards L, Brown CB. Icodextrin 7.5% dialysate solution (glucose polymer) in patients with ultrafiltration failure: extension of CAPD technique survival. *Perit Dial Int* 1997;17: 84–7.

9   Twardowski ZJ, Nolph KD, Khanna R *et al.* Peritoneal Equilibration Test. *Perit Dial Bull* 1987;7:138–47.

10 Korbet SM, Roxby RM. Peritoneal membrane failure: differential diagnosis – evaluation and treatment. *Semin Dial* 1994;7:128–37.

11 Rocco MV, Jordan JR, Burkart JM. Changes in peritoneal transport during the first month of peritoneal dialysis. *Perit Dial Int* 1995;15:12-17.

12   Davies SJ, Coles GA, Topley N. Problems of peritoneal membrane failure. In: Mehta A, Lameire NH (eds). *Complications of dialysis – recognition and management*. New York: Marcel Dekker, 2000:151–78.

13   Ho-dac-Pannekeet MM, Atasever B, Struijk DG, Krediet RT. Analysis of ultrafiltration failure in peritoneal dialysis patients by means of standard peritoneal permeability analysis. *Perit Dial Int* 1997;**17**:144–50.

14   Heaf J. CAPD adequacy and dialysis morbidity: detrimental effect of a high peritoneal equilibration rate. *Ren Fail* 1995;**17**:575–87.

15   Churchill DN, Thorpe KE, Nolph KD *et al*. Increased peritoneal membrane transport is associated with decreased patient and technique survival for continuous peritoneal dialysis patients. *J Am Soc Nephrol* 1998;**9**:1285–92.

16   Davies SJ, Phillips L, Russell GI. Peritoneal solute transport predicts survival on CAPD independently of residual renal function. *Nephrol Dial Transplant* 1998;**13**:962–8.

17   Coles GA. Have we underestimated the importance of fluid balance for the survival of PD patients? [editorial]. *Perit Dial Int* 1997;**17**:321–6.

18   Churchill DN, Taylor DW, Keshaviah PR. Adequacy of dialysis and nutrition in continuous peritoneal dialysis: association with clinical outcome. *J Am Soc Nephrol* 1996;**7**:198–207.

19   Davies SJ, Phillips L, Griffiths AM *et al*. What really happens to people on long-term peritoneal dialysis? *Kidney Int* 1998;**54**:2207–17.

20   Maiorca R, Cancarini GC, Zubani R *et al*. CAPD viability: a long-term comparison with hemodialysis. *Perit Dial Int* 1996;**16**:276–87.

21   Maiorca R, Brunori G, Zubani R *et al*. Predictive value of dialysis adequacy and nutritional indices for mortality and morbidity in CAPD and HD patients. A longitudinal study. *Nephrol Dial Transplant* 1995;**10**:2295–2305.

22   Selgas RB, Fernandez-Reyes MA, Bosque MJ *et al*. An analysis of adequacy of dialysis in a selected population on CAPD ever three years: The influence of urea and creatinine kinetics. *Nephrol Dial Transplant* 1993;**8**:1244–53.

23   Lamiere NH, Vanholder R, Van Loo A *et al*. Cardiovascular diseases in peritoneal dialysis patients: the size of the problem. *Kidney Int* 1996;**50**:S28–36.

24   Davies SJ, Phillips L, Griffiths AM *et al*. Impact of peritoneal membrane function on long-term clinical outcome in peritoneal dialysis patients. *Perit Dial Int* 1999;**19**(Suppl 2):S91–4.

25   Amann K, Mandelbaum A, Schwarz U, Ritz E. Hypertension and left ventricular hypertrophy in the CAPD patient. *Kidney Int* 1996;**50**(Suppl. 56):S37–40.

26   Mujais S, Nolph K, Gokal R *et al*. Evaluation and management of ultrafiltration problems in peritoneal dialysis. International Society for Peritoneal Dialysis Ad Hoc Committee on Ultrafiltration Management in Peritoneal Dialysis. *Perit Dial Int* 2000;**20**(Suppl 4):S5–21.

27   Posthuma N, ter Wee PM, Verbrugh HA *et al*. Icodextrin instead of glucose during the daytime dwell in CCPD increases ultrafiltration and 24-h dialysate creatinine clearance. *Nephrol Dial Transplant* 1997;**12**:550–3.

28   Woodrow G, Oldroyd B, Stables G *et al*. Effects of icodextrin in automated peritoneal dialysis on blood pressure and bioelectrical impedance analysis. *Nephrol Dial Transplant* 2000;**15**:862–6.

29   National Kidney Foundation. NKF-DOQI clinical practice guidelines for peritoneal dialysis adequacy. *Am J Kidney Dis* 1997;**30**:S67–136.

30   Blake PG. Problems predicting continuous ambulatory peritoneal dialysis outcomes with small solute clearances. *Perit Dial Int* 1993;**13**(Suppl 2):S209–11.

31   Genestier S, Hedelin G, Schaffer P, Faller B. Prognostic factors in CAPD patients: a retrospective study of a 10-year period. *Nephrol Dial Transplant* 1995;**10**:1905–11.

32   Churchill DN, Blake P, Goldstein MB *et al* and Canadian Society of Nephrology Committee for Clinical Practice Guidelines. Clinical Practice Guidelines of the Canadian Society of Nephrology for treatment of patients with chronic renal failure. *J Am Soc Nephrol* 1999;**10**(Suppl 13):S287–S321.

33 Blake PG. Adequacy of peritoneal dialysis. *Curr Opin Nephrol Hypertens* 1996;**5**:492–6.

34 Burkart JM, Schreiber M, Korbet SM *et al*. Solute clearance approach to adequacy of peritoneal dialysis. *Perit Dial Int* 1996;**16**:457–70.

35 Vonesh EF, Burkart J, McMurray SD, Williams PF. Peritoneal dialysis kinetic modeling: validation in a multicenter clinical study. *Perit Dial Int* 1996;**16**:471–81.

36 Gokal R, Harty J. Are there limits for CAPD? Adequacy and nutritional considerations [editorial]. *Perit Dial Int* 1996;**16**:437–41.

37 Pamagua R, Amato D, Vonesh E *et al*. Effects of increased peritoneal clearances on mortality rates in peritoneal dialysis: ADEMEX, a prospective, randomised, controlled trial. *J Am Soc Nephrol* 2002;**13**:1307–20.

38 Harty JC, Boulton H, Curwell J *et al*. The normalized protein catabolic rate is a flawed marker of nutrition in CAPD patients. *Kidney Int* 1994;**45**:103–9.

39 Davies SJ, Phillips L, Griffiths AM *et al*. Analysis of the effects of increasing delivered dialysis treatment to malnourished peritoneal dialysis patients. *Kidney Int* 2000;**57**:1743–54.

40 Mak SK, Wong PN, Lo KY *et al*. Randomized prospective study of the effect of increased dialytic dose on nutritional and clinical outcome in continuous ambulatory peritoneal dialysis patients. *Am J Kidney Dis* 2000;**36**:105–14.

41 Tattersall JE, Doyle S, Greenwood RN, Farrington K. Kinetic modelling and underdialysis in CAPD patients. *Nephrol Dial Transplant* 1993;**8**:535–8.

42 Metcalf JE, Harris KPG, Walls J. Role of diurectics in the preservation of residual renal function in patients on continuous ambulatory peritoneal dialysis. *Kidney Int* 2001;**59**:1128–33.

43 Port FK, Held PJ, Nolph KD *et al*. Risk of peritonitis and technique failure by CAPD connection technique: a national study. *Kidney Int* 1992;**42**:967–74.

44 Working Party of British Society of Antimicrobial Chemotherapy (BSAC). Diagnosis and management of peritonitis in CAPD. *Lancet* 1987;**i**:845–8.

45 Keane WF, Alexander SR, Bailie GR *et al*. Peritoneal dialysis-related peritonitis treatment recommendations: 1996 update. *Perit Dial Int* 1996;**16**:557–73.

46 Golper TA, Tranaeus A. Vancomycin revisited. *Perit Dial Int* 1996;**16**:116–7.

47 Keane WF, Bailie GR, Boeschoten E *et al*. Adult peritoneal dialysis-related peritonitis treatment recommendations: 2000 update. *Perit Dial Int* 2000;**20**:396–411.

48 Gokal R, Alexander S, Ash S *et al*. Peritoneal catheters and exit-site practices toward optimum peritoneal access: 1998 update. (Official report from the International Society for Peritoneal Dialysis). *Perit Dial Int* 1998;**18**:11–33.

49 Holley JL, Piraino B, Dacko C *et al*. Managing *Staphylococcus aureus* catheter infection in continuous ambulatory peritoneal dialysis patients. *Adv Ren Replace Ther* 1994;**1**:167–75.

50 Luzar MA, Coles GA, Faller B *et al*. *Staphylococcus aureus* nasal carriage and infection in patients on continuous ambulatory peritoneal dialysis. *N Engl J Med* 1990;**322**:505–09.

51 Piraino B. *Staphylococcus aureus* infections in dialysis patients: focus on prevention. *ASAIO J* 2000;**46**:S13–7.

52 Bernardini J, Piraino B, Holley J *et al*. A randomized trial of *Staphylococcus aureus* prophylaxis in peritoneal dialysis patients: mupirocin calcium ointment 2% applied to the exit site versus cyclic oral rifampin. *Am J Kidney Dis* 1996;**27**:695–700.

53 Vas SI, Conly J, Bargman JM, Oreopoulos DG. Resistance to mupirocin: no indication of it to date while using mupirocin ointment for prevention of *Staphylococcus aureus* exit-site infections in peritoneal dialysis patients [editorial]. *Perit Dial Int* 1999;**19**:313–14.

54 Watson AR, Gartland G on behalf of the European Paediatric Peritoneal Working Group. Guidelines by an *ad hoc* European committee on elective peritoneal dialysis in pediatric patients. *Perit Dial Int* 2001;**21**:240–4.

55 Coleman JE, Edefonti A, Watson AR. Guidelines by an *ad hoc* European committee on the assessment of growth and nutritional status in children on chronic peritoneal dialysis. *Perit Dial Int* 2001;**21**:323.

56 Kari JA, Gonzalez C, Lederman SE *et al*. Outcome and growth of infants with severe chronic renal failure. *Kidney Int* 2000;**57**:1681–7.

57 Schroder CH. The choice of dialysis solutions in pediatric peritoneal dialysis: guidelines by an *ad hoc* Europen committee. *Perit Dial Int* 2001;**21**:568–74.

58 Ansell D, Feest T (eds). The UK Renal Registry. *The second annual report*, 1999. Bristol: UK Renal Registry, 1999;175–87.

59 Schaefer F. Adequacy of peritoneal dialysis in children. In: Fine RN, Alexander SR, Warady BA (eds). *CAPD/CCPD in children*, 2nd edn. Boston: Kluwer Academic Publishers, 1998:99–118.

60 Morgenstern B. Structure and function of the pediatric peritoneal membrane. In: Fine RN, Alexander SR, Warady BA (eds). *CAPD/CCPD in children*, 2nd edn. Boston: Kluwer Academic Publishers, 1998:73–86.

61 Fischbach M, Terzic J, Bergere V *et al*. The optimal approach to peritoneal dialysis prescription in children. *Perit Dial Int* 1999;**19**:S474–8.

62 Fischbach M, Stefandis C, Watson AR. Guidelines by an *ad hoc* European committee on adequacy of the pediatric peritoneal dialysis prescription. *Nephrol Dial Transplant* 2002;**17**:380–5.

63 National Kidney Foundation. NKF-DOQI clinical practice guidelines for peritoneal dialysis adequacy. *Am J Kidney Dis* 1997;**30**:S67–136.

64 Holtta T, Ronnholm K, Jalanko H, Holmberg C. Clinical outcome of pediatric patients on peritoneal dialysis under adequacy control. *Pediatr Nephrol* 2000;14:889–98.

65 Edefonti A, Verrina E, Schaefer F *et al*. The European experience with CAPD/CCPD in children. In: Fine RN, Alexander SR, Warady BA (eds). *CAPD/CCPD in children*, 2nd edn. Boston: Kluwer Academic Publishers, 1998;17–34.

66 Klaus G, Schaefer F, Muller-Wiefel D, Mehls O and members of APN. Treatment of peritoneal dialysis-associated peritonitis with continuous versus intermittent vancomycin/teicoplanin and ceftazidime in children: preliminary results of a prospective randomised trial. *Adv Perit Dial* 1995;**11**:296–301.

67 Gokal R, Alexander S, Ash S *et al*. Peritoneal catheters and exit-site practices toward optimum peritoneal access: 1998 update. *Perit Dial Int* 1998;**18**:11–33.

68 Alexander SR, Donaldson LA, Sullivan KE. CAPD/CCPD for children in North America: The NAPRTCS experience. In: Fine RN, Alexander SR, Warady BA (eds). *CAPD/CCPD in children*, 2nd edn. Boston: Kluwer Academic Publishers, 1998;5–8.

69 Arbeiter K, Pichler A, Muerwald G *et al*. Timing of peritoneal dialysis catheter removal after pediatric renal transplantation. *Perit Dial Int* 2001;**21**:467–70.

5 Haemodialysis and peritoneal dialysis: nutritional and biochemical standards

Introduction

5.1 Renal failure has major adverse effects on the body's chemistry which are, in part, corrected by dialysis. In attempting to maintain satisfactory blood chemistry, dietary restrictions are also necessary. Maintaining optimal nutrition and achieving good biochemical control are, therefore, important aspects in the management of patients on dialysis.

Blood sampling

5.2 All blood samples from haemodialysis (HD) patients should be taken on a mid-week dialysis, ie after the 'short gap'. Clinicians should be aware that some abnormalities, eg of serum potassium, will be more severe after the 'long gap'.

Albumin

Recommendation

▶ Serum albumin should be measured regularly. A serum albumin concentration below 35 g/l, using a Bromocresol Green assay, or below 30 g/l using a Bromocresol Purple assay, should prompt clinical reassessment of the patient, looking for fluid overload, malnutrition, underdialysis, and remediable causes of an acute phase response. No audit standards can be set for measurements of serum albumin until there has been progress in standardisation of assays between different laboratories and in the understanding of the causes and appropriate treatment of hypoalbuminaemia in dialysis patients. (**Good practice**)

RATIONALE

5.3 Hypoalbuminaemia is an adverse prognostic marker for survival in patients on dialysis and after renal transplantation.[1–9] Possible causes include malnutrition, dilution as a result of salt and water overload,[10] increased peritoneal losses during peritoneal dialysis (PD),[11] increased transcapillary escape and, perhaps most importantly, an inflammatory response.[12] Serum albumin concentration, however, is a very unreliable marker of nutritional status.[12,13] Recently, a close correlation between hypoalbuminaemia and markers of the acute phase response, such as C-reactive protein (CRP), has been shown,[14–17] suggesting that chronic inflammation may contribute to the excess mortality possibly by accelerating atherosclerosis or exacerbating heart failure. Persistent elevation of CRP is common in dialysis patients, and may occur in the absence of detectable infection.

5.4 An increase in mean dialysis dose has been reported to increase mean serum albumin in one single-centre study,[18] but this increase was achieved by conversion to more bio-compatible membranes, and may therefore have improved serum albumin not by improving nutritional status, but by removing a cause of chronic inflammation. There are few data to show that dietary intervention or alteration of dialysis or drug prescription can correct hypoalbuminaemia in dialysis patients; one recent randomised trial,[19] however, has shown a significant rise in serum albumin after three months of treatment with oral essential amino acids. Inclusion of serum albumin as an audit measure would only be justified if it were clear how clinicians should react to hypoalbuminaemia to close the audit loop. It is recommended that data on serum albumin should, however, continue to be collected, to allow identification of high risk patients.

5.5   An additional difficulty is the variation in assays used. The Bromocresol Green assay may over-estimate true serum albumin concentration by up to 5 g/l, but uraemic serum may interfere in the Bromocresol Purple method, causing under-estimation of true serum albumin concentration by around 7 g/l.[20,21] The reference range quoted by different UK laboratories using the same assay varies considerably, being derived either from the manufacturer, local studies, or textbooks: the proportion of patients with a serum albumin within the reference range in a given unit is therefore mostly determined by how low the lower limit of normal is set, and may not reflect any real difference between that and another unit where the reference range is different.[22] There is a pressing need for standardisation of measurement of serum albumin or for wholesale conversion to more reliable assays.

Bicarbonate

Recommendations

▶ Serum bicarbonate, before a HD session, measured with minimal delay after venepuncture should be between 20 and 26 mmol/l. **(C)**

▶ For continuous ambulatory peritoneal dialysis (CAPD) patients serum bicarbonate, measured with minimal delay after venepuncture, should be between 25 and 29 mmol/l. **(B)**

RATIONALE

5.6   Interpretation of the relationship between serum bicarbonate and outcome in dialysis patients is complicated because a low pre-dialysis serum bicarbonate may reflect either inadequate correction of acidosis by dialysis or a high protein intake. Experimental and clinical studies have shown that acidosis increases protein catabolism in dialysis patients, and that correction of acidosis by adjustment of dialysate bicarbonate concentration and/or by sodium bicarbonate supplementation results in less protein catabolism.[23] Control of acidosis has not been shown to improve outcome. More aggressive correction of pre-dialysis acidosis could conceivably do harm by several mechanisms:

1   Sodium bicarbonate may contribute to sodium retention and thus to volume expansion and to hypertension.

2   Alkalosis decreases the solubility of calcium phosphate and thus may increase the risk of extra-articular and vascular calcification.[23]

3   Alkalosis shifts phosphate into cells and thus may impair dialytic phosphate removal and result in post-dialysis rebound hyperphosphataemia.

4   Alkalosis may cause hypoventilation during dialysis, which may contribute to cardiovascular instability during dialysis.

5.7   An additional difficulty is in the measurement of serum bicarbonate. Measured serum or plasma bicarbonate values fall over time following venepuncture, and this may result in systematically lower bicarbonate levels in patients whose samples have to be transported to a central laboratory prior to analysis, for example from satellite dialysis units. This problem of falsely low bicarbonate levels is particularly associated with under-filled or uncapped sample tubes and prolonged storage of samples at room temperature.[24] The previous edition of this document set a standard that for HD patients, pre-dialysis bicarbonate concentration should be within the local laboratory reference range in all patients who had been on HD for longer than three months. However, data from the Renal Registry[22] show that the degree of compliance with this target in each centre correlates closely with the lower limit of the reference range bicarbonate in the laboratory or laboratories used by that centre. The lower the limit, the more patients fall within the standard.

5.8   Lowrie and Lew reported significantly higher death rates, after adjustment for other laboratory variables and case mix (but not dialysis dose), in HD patients with pre-dialysis serum bicarbonate less than 12.5 mmol/l and above 20 mmol/l, compared with the reference group of 17.5–20 mmol/l.[25] Such observational studies cannot, however, differentiate between the beneficial effects of higher dietary intake of protein against the potentially deleterious effects of incomplete correction of acidosis by dialysis. No intervention studies have examined the effect of different degrees of correction of pre-dialysis acidosis on morbidity or mortality in HD patients. In a study of 200 CAPD patients randomised to high or standard bicarbonate dialysate, with supplemental oral sodium bicarbonate and calcium carbonate in the high bicarbonate group, Stein *et al*[26] showed significantly fewer hospital admissions in the high bicarbonate group. While awaiting further such trials, it is believed that the benefits of correction of acidosis on muscle and bone metabolism outweigh any likely adverse effects. A lower standard is set for HD than for PD patients because serum bicarbonate is at its lowest when measured immediately prior to HD.

Parathyroid hormone

Standard

▶ Parathyroid hormone (PTH) concentrations should be less than four times the upper limit of normal of the assay used in patients being managed for chronic renal failure or after transplantation and in patients who have been on HD or PD for longer than three months. **(B)**

RATIONALE

5.9   There is convincing evidence of bone resistance to the effects of PTH in patients with chronic renal failure (CRF) and those on dialysis: normal bone turnover is associated with a PTH concentration four times normal in chronic renal failure and three times normal in dialysis patients. Some recommend that PTH should be maintained at 3–4 times the upper limit (using an assay for the intact PTH molecule) of the non-renal normal range in order to ensure normal bone turnover. Low bone turnover is associated with hypercalcaemia and, possibly, an increased risk of fracture and vascular calcification. Low calcium dialysate can be used to stimulate parathyroid activity. There is a danger, however, that failure to suppress secondary hyperparathyroidism fully will permit progressive parathyroid hyperplasia, leading to severe hyperparathyroid bone disease and the need for surgical parathyroidectomy, particularly in patients with slowly progressive pre-end stage renal disease (ESRD). Also, raised PTH concentrations may be responsible for increased cardiac calcium content, vascular calcification, and insulin resistance associated with secondary hyperparathyroidism. The relative importance of hyperparathyroidism as a risk factor for premature vascular disease in renal failure is difficult to determine from observational studies, and no informative randomised controlled trials exist. Some evidence is available linking hyperparathyroidism with valvular calcification, vascular calcification, and calciphylaxis. However, phosphate retention is a cause both of hyperparathyroidism and of pathological calcification, and the exact role of raised PTH levels and phosphate retention remains uncertain. Some evidence suggests that low bone turnover, associated with low PTH levels, may be directly associated with an increased risk of vascular calcification and other cardiovascular complications.[27] In the absence of firm evidence, individual clinicians should decide on the degree to which hyperparathyroidism should be corrected, and on how this should be achieved. There is no doubt, however, that a parathyroid hormone concentration over four times the upper limit of normal is associated with an increased risk of significant bone disease, and that this should therefore be avoided by medical (or if necessary surgical) treatment of hyperparathyroidism.

5.10 A small proportion of patients will have such significant co-morbidity and limited life expectancy that their physicians will choose to ignore asymptomatic hyperparathyroidism. At any time, a significant proportion of patients on dialysis will be new entrants to the dialysis programme, up to 45% of whom will not have received nephrological care for more than three months prior to inception of dialysis.[28]

Phosphate

5.11 Hyperphosphataemia is common in dialysis patients and contributes to the pathogenesis of hyperparathyroidism;[29] adequate control of serum phosphate may therefore be necessary for control of hyperparathyroidism. Together with hyperparathyroidism, hyperphosphataemia and/or a raised calcium phosphate product are also risk factors for vascular calcification, calcification of the aortic and mitral valve rings[30-4] and peri-articular calcification. The effects of standard HD on serum phosphate are limited, due to the high distribution volume, which leads to rapid rebound of serum phosphate after dialysis. However, daily HD results in normalisation of phosphate concentrations, and even hypophosphataemia. Hyperphosphataemia can be controlled in the majority of patients by the use of phosphate binders taken with meals. A variety of phosphate binders are available, including aluminium hydroxide, calcium carbonate, calcium acetate, and sevelamer hydrochloride. The choice of agents should be individualised, as all currently available agents carry different cost:benefit and risk:benefit ratios. For instance, calcium salts may promote positive calcium balance and result in vascular calcification. Long-term use of aluminium salts may contribute to intellectual deterioration and to other features of aluminium toxicity.[35,36] Aluminium hydroxide should only be used where the benefit of achieving improved phosphate control is judged likely to outweigh this risk.

5.12   Interpretation of serum pre-dialysis phosphate levels is difficult because phosphate intake often mirrors protein intake; low serum phosphate may be a surrogate for undernutrition, and vice versa. This type of 'confounding by reverse causality', when a putative risk factor is influenced by another risk factor, complicates any attempt to derive evidence-based standards from observational data on the relationship between serum phosphate and outcome.

5.13   Several studies have examined the predictive effect of serum phosphate on subsequent mortality. Lowrie and Lew found a U-shaped relationship between serum phosphate measured at the beginning of 1989 and mortality over the subsequent 12 months, after adjustment for age, sex, race, diabetes, primary renal disease, and time on dialysis. The relative risk of death associated with a low serum phosphate was less after statistical adjustment for other laboratory variables, but the risk of mortality with a high serum phosphate was higher after adjustment.[25] A Japanese study of 1,982 new dialysis patients found no relationship between serum phosphate taken immediately prior to inception of dialysis, and mortality,[37] but no information was given about the patients established on dialysis. A further study showed a difference in mortality between the lowest three quintiles of serum phosphate (in mmol/l) (0.35–1.42, 1.45–1.78, 1.81–2.10) and the two quintiles with serum phosphate (2.13–2.52 and 2.55–5.46).[38] The authors concluded that serum phosphate should be maintained below 2.1 mmol/l. Similar conclusions were reached on analysis of data from the UK Renal Registry.[22] A recent study, not yet published in full, reported on 40,538 prevalent HD patients with at least one measurement of pre-dialysis serum calcium and phosphate in the last quarter of 1997. After adjustment for numerous covariates including markers of nutritional status and dialysis dose, there was a progressive increase in relative risk of death as phosphate rose. In the population as a whole and in each category of serum phosphate, mortality also increased with rising serum calcium concentrations.[39]

5.14   Normalisation of serum phosphate in patients receiving thrice weekly HD in the UK is very difficult, as shown by the low proportion of patients achieving the standard of less than 1.7 mmol/l in the third report of the Renal Registry.[22]

Calcium

Standard

▶ Serum calcium, adjusted for albumin concentration, should be between 2.2 and 2.6 mmol/l, in HD (pre-dialysis sample) patients and in PD patients. **(B)**

RATIONALE

5.15   Reasons for controlling serum calcium include the need to prevent stimulation of parathyroid gland activity by hypocalcaemia and the need to prevent symptomatic hypercalcaemia. Serum calcium is determined by dietary intake, including the intake of calcium-based phosphate binders, and by dialysate calcium. In patients with secondary hyperparathyroidism, it may be preferable to maintain serum calcium towards the top of the normal range; in patients with low bone turnover, a relatively low serum calcium may help to promote bone turnover, and low calcium dialysate may be used to achieve this. Severe hypercalcaemia (>3.0 mmol/l) was associated with increased mortality in a case-mix adjusted study.[25] Some found no relationship between serum calcium and survival in their series, followed for 3–32 years,[37] while others showed that a low adjusted serum calcium level was independently predictive of death in HD patients, and that chronic hypocalcaemia was associated both with ischaemic heart disease and cardiac failure.[40] In contrast, another large study found that the relative risk of death, adjusted for multiple covariates, increased with rising serum calcium.[39] Estimation of serum calcium, corrected for albumin, is susceptible to all the problems with inter-assay variation (see section on albumin). In addition, there are numerous formulae in use for 'correction' of serum calcium for albumin concentration. Comparison of standards of care between units, with regard to control of serum calcium will, therefore, remain difficult until these problems have been resolved. The UK Renal Registry will continue to collect the raw data on serum albumin and total serum calcium, adjust for inter-assay variations in albumin assay, and apply a standard formula. In the longer term, it would be desirable for units managing renal patients to have access to reliable direct assays for ionised calcium.

Potassium

Standard

▶ Pre-dialysis serum potassium should be between 3.5 and 6.5 mmol/l in HD patients. Serum potassium should be between 3.5 and 5.5 mmol/l in PD patients. (**Good practice**)

RATIONALE

5.16   Hyperkalaemia is an important potential cause of sudden death in dialysis patients. It decreases cardiac and neuromuscular excitability, and may cause sudden death from asystole. Hypokalaemia increases the risk of cardiac arrythmias, particularly in patients on digoxin. A U-shaped relationship between pre-dialysis serum potassium concentration and relative risk of death has been described in one large study.[25]

5.17   Although no standard has been set for post-dialysis measurements, severe hypokalaemia post-dialysis should be avoided. Although it may be necessary, in some patients (eg those with recurrent pre-dialysis hyperkalaemia), to utilise low potassium dialysate to maximise potassium removal, it would be preferable to concentrate on reduction of dietary potassium intake and the avoidance of drugs which might contribute to pre-dialysis hyperkalaemia, including angiotensin converting enzyme (ACE) inhibitors (which decrease colonic potassium secretion).

Aluminium

Recommendation

▶ Serum aluminium concentration should be measured every three months in all patients on HD and in all PD patients receiving oral aluminium hydroxide. No patient whose ferritin level is <100 µg/l should have a serum aluminium concentration >60 µg/l (2.2 µmol/l). (**B**)

RATIONALE

5.18   Aluminium can accumulate in patients on dialysis either as a result of inadequate removal of aluminium from mains water used to prepare dialysate, or as a result of gastrointestinal absorption of aluminium in patients prescribed aluminium hydroxide as a dietary phosphate binder. Aluminium accumulation can cause anaemia, severe bone disease, and encephalopathy. It is therefore mandatory to monitor patients at risk for evidence of aluminium accumulation. Patients at risk include all those on HD, whether in centres or at home, and all patients prescribed oral aluminium salts as dietary phosphate binders. Patients receiving other aluminium-containing drugs such as antacids, particularly if used in combination with citrate salts, which increase bio-availability of aluminium, should also be screened. (Patients prescribed aluminium salts should be warned to avoid taking these with fruit juices or other sources of citric or ascorbic acid.) Serum levels reflect current exposure, and if measured regularly should permit identification of patients undergoing excessive exposure, but do not reflect cumulative aluminium burden, assessment of which requires desferrioxamine tests or bone biopsy. Serum levels depend on the amount of free transferrin available, and may therefore be increased in the presence of relative iron deficiency; patients with serum ferritin below 100 g/l whose serum aluminium levels are above 60 g/l (2.2 mol/l) should therefore be re-investigated after iron repletion. Aluminium can be removed safely from dialysate water, the type of water treatment being dependent on the mains water aluminium level. Oral aluminium salts continue to be used to control phosphate accumulation in dialysis patients. Whether such use is a significant risk factor for aluminium toxicity is less certain than is the case for contamination of dialysate, but at least one study has shown a correlation between cumulative dosage of aluminium hydroxide and intellectual deterioration. Such risks, however, need to be weighed against the risk of phosphate retention and against the risks, and costs, of alternative strategies to control serum phosphate.

Further guidelines for the investigation and management of patients with possible aluminium accumulation were published as a result of a consensus conference held in 1992.[41]

Nutritional screening

Standard

▶ All patients with ESRD both before and after the start of dialysis should undergo regular screening for undernutrition. (**Good practice**)

Recommendations

▶ Nutritional screening should include as a minimum subjective global assessment (SGA) measurement of height, weight and serum albumin. Body mass index (BMI) should be calculated (weight in kilograms divided by the square of the height in metres) and unintentional loss of oedema free weight recorded. (**Good practice**)

▶ A diagnosis of undernutrition should be considered if any one of the following criteria are met:

- BMI <18.5
- unintentional loss of oedema free weight >10% in past six months
- albumin <35 g/l (Bromocresol Green) or <30 g/l (Bromocresol Purple) (**B**)
- SGA scores of 1–2 (severe undernutrition) or 3–5 (mild to moderate undernutrition). (**Good practice**)

RATIONALE

5.19   Both low pre-dialysis serum creatinine concentrations and low serum cholesterol concentrations at the start of renal replacement therapy are highly predictive of poor outcome.[1,3,8,25,27,42–4] These associations are probably due to the deleterious effects of malnutrition. There is no single 'gold standard' measurement of undernutrition. This has led to the recommendation that a panel of measurements be used which reflect the various aspects of protein-calorie nutrition.[45] In this document an approach has been used which combines both subjective global assessment and techniques recently developed by the Malnutrition Advisory Group (MAG) of the British Association for Parenteral and Enteral Nutrition (BAPEN).[46] This uses a small number of measurements with well defined cut-off values. BMI is a simple, accurate and reproducible measurement. Its calculation from height and weight is automatically provided in most renal computer systems. We have employed a cut-off which in the UK has a Z-score of 2 (2 standard deviation scores below the median) in the normal population. A similar cut-off has been proposed by the World Health Organization (WHO)[47] and is associated with adverse functional outcome measurements. It is recognised that a few healthy individuals may have a BMI less than 18.5. In patients with CRF the presence of oedema may lead to an overestimate of the BMI and where possible the oedema free weight should be recorded. Unintentional loss of oedema free weight of greater than 10% in six months is associated with functional abnormalities and poor clinical outcome in the general population.[48] It is well recognised that hypoalbuminaemia is a powerful predictor of morbidity and mortality in patients with ESRD although factors other than nutritional intake are known to decrease serum albumin and thus affect its specificity. SGA has been widely used in nutritional surveys in patients with CRF.[49] A score is derived from subjective and objective aspects of the medical history and physical examination[50] which allows patients to be categorised as having either normal, mild, moderate or severe malnutrition.

Assessment of nutritional status in undernourished patients

Recommendation

▶ If a diagnosis of undernutrition is suspected on the above criteria then a full nutritional assessment should be undertaken by a clinician and renal dietitian to elucidate the underlying cause. This should include a full medical history, assessment of dietary intake (three-day dietary record and measurement of the protein equivalent of nitrogen appearance), measurement of CRP, serum bicarbonate and measurement of dialysis adequacy and residual renal function. **(Good practice)**

RATIONALE

5.20   Many factors predispose to the development of undernutrition in patients with CRF. Some, such as changes in appetite, dental problems, vomiting and diarrhoea, may be identified through the patient's medical history. A decrease in appetite secondary to either uraemia or underdialysis should be confirmed with an assessment of dietary intake. This can be obtained indirectly through the normalised equivalent of total protein nitrogen appearance (PNA) although this may give a spuriously high estimate in the presence of weight loss or active catabolism. A variety of techniques are available for recording dietary intake; food intake records and dietary recall are the commonest. The dietary protein intake in pre-dialysis patients who are not being prescribed a low protein intake should be at least 0.75 g kg^{-1} day^{-1}; in HD and PD patients it should be at least 1.2 g kg^{-1} day^{-1}. Dietary energy intake in all three groups should be at least 35 kcal/kg/day, although 30 kcal/kg/day may be sufficient in those over the age of 60. In pre-dialysis patients it has been shown that dietary protein intake spontaneously decreases with decreasing glomerular filtration rate (GFR).[51,52] That undernutrition may be associated with an inflammatory state is well recognised and a persistently elevated CRP level will suggest this diagnosis.[53,54] Acidosis is a well established catabolic factor[55] and to minimise this the bicarbonate concentration of CAPD and HD patients should be maintained within the ranges stated in the preceding section.

Management of malnutrition

Recommendations

▶ In all patients found to have an inadequate dietary intake, identifiable causes should be corrected and dietary advice given to increase intake. Oral supplements, intraperitoneal amino acids (IPAA – CAPD), intradialytic parenteral nutrition (IDPN – HD), nasogastric (NG) feeding, percutaneous endoscopic gastrostomy (PEG) feeding and intravenous partial/total parenteral nutrition are all recognised means by which dietary intake can be supplemented. Local protocols incorporating these methods should be agreed. **(Good practice)**

▶ In those patients found to have a persistently high CRP, a source of infection should be sought and treated. **(Good practice)**

▶ Where dietary intake is adequate, catabolic factors such as acidosis, thyrotoxicosis and uncontrolled diabetes should be sought and treated. **(Good practice)**

RATIONALE

5.21   Various factors including uraemia, depression, gastroparesis, cancer, heart failure and anorexia nervosa are associated with a low dietary intake. Oral supplements should be tried initially although their efficacy has been shown to be greatest in those with a BMI <20.[56] Failing this, both IPAA and IDPN have been shown to be beneficial in PD and HD patients.[57,58] NG feeding, although effective in the hospitalised patient, is not so well tolerated by outpatients and in this group a PEG should be considered, although for this it may be necessary to transfer PD patients to HD.

Dietary sodium intake

Recommendation

▶ All patients with ESRD both before and after the start of dialysis should be advised to limit dietary salt intake to less than 6 g/day (equivalent to approximately 100 mmol of sodium). **(B)**

RATIONALE

5.22   The reference nutrient intake (two standard deviations above the estimated average requirement) for sodium intake in adults in the UK is 70 mmol/day.[59] The average intake of the population is substantially greater than this. Although the beneficial effects of dietary sodium restriction on hypertension have been disputed,[60] there is substantial evidence to suggest that a reduction in dietary sodium intake in the normal population results in a reduction in blood pressure over and above that seen with a 'healthy' diet.[61,62] Similar results have been obtained in HD patients[63] in combination with a low sodium dialysate.

Obesity

Recommendation

▶ All patients with CRF should receive dietary advice to avoid weight gain beyond a BMI >30. **(C)**

RATIONALE

5.23 Overweight levels are graded by the WHO according to BMI whereby grade 1 overweight is 25.00–29.99, grade 2 is 30.00–39.99 and grade 3 is ≥40.[64] Within the general population, both gaining weight to become overweight and being overweight are associated with increased morbidity and mortality. There are, however, no long-term intervention studies that show that sustained weight loss is associated with a decrease in morbidity and mortality. Within the HD population, the lowest mortality is seen in those patients with the highest BMI.[65] An explanation for this might be that in this group being overweight is accompanied by better nutrition,[66] the beneficial effects of this outweighing any adverse effects of being overweight. There are no intervention studies that have examined either gaining or losing weight to or from an overweight state respectively in dialysis patients.

Paediatric section

Parathyroid hormone (PTH), phosphate and calcium

Standard

▶ Serum phosphate and calcium should be kept within the normal range. PTH levels should be maintained within twice the upper limit of the normal range but, contrary to adult standards, may be kept within the normal range if growth is normal. **(B)**

RATIONALE

5.24 Phosphate values (mmol/l) are variable throughout childhood; 50th centile (±2 SD) is 1.85 (1.4–2.3) at birth, falling to 1.7 (1.2–2.1) at six months, 1.55 (1.1–1.95) at one year, and 1.4 (1.05–1.75) at three years and remaining fairly constant thereafter throughout childhood. Control of serum phosphate is essential to prevent hyperparathyroidism, and can usually be achieved through dietary restriction and the use of phosphate binders. Serum calcium levels vary less throughout childhood and should be kept in the normal range. Dietary assessment to ensure adequate calcium intake is recommended.

5.25 PTH should be measured early in the course of CRF, as levels may rise in advance of any abnormalities in serum phosphate or calcium concentration.[67] There is no evidence in childhood to suggest an optimal level for the maintenance of PTH. Consequently there is no universal agreement as to whether PTH levels should be maintained within the normal range or within twice the normal range in order to prevent adynamic bone disease, which may adversely affect growth.

Nutritional management and growth

Standards

▶ Measures of supine length or standing height and weight should be monitored at each clinic visit. Head circumference should be measured at each visit before two years of age and six monthly up to five years of age. All measurements should be plotted on reference European growth charts for healthy children.[68] The data should be returned to the UK Renal Registry every six months. (**Good practice**)

▶ All children should undergo dietary assessment by a paediatric renal dietitian at a minimum of every three months, but more often if there is deteriorating biochemistry or growth. Inadequate intake should be supplemented orally or enterally. (**Good practice**)

▶ Recombinant human growth hormone (rhGH) may be offered to children of all ages who have a height standard deviation score (Ht SDS) more than 2 SD below the mean (or below the 2nd percentile), and a height velocity SDS less than the 25th centile, whose growth has failed to respond to adequate nutrition, correction of metabolic abnormalities, adequate dialysis and, if post transplant, reduction of prednisolone to a minimum. (**B**)

RATIONALE

5.26 Input from a paediatric renal dietitian is crucial to prescribe, monitor and maintain satisfactory standards of nutritional care for each child because of the changing needs for growth and development.[69] Energy intakes need to be maximised, with some children requiring an energy supplement. The oral route is always the first choice for delivery of the nutritional prescription. Delivery of supplementary feeding using nasogastric or gastrostomy tubes should be considered when the child's oral intake fails to meet recommended nutritional intakes and/or the child fails to maintain an adequate growth velocity, especially in young infants.[70] Protein and phosphate intakes should be moderated on an individual basis.

5.27 The nutritional status of children should be evaluated before commencing dialysis and preferably at monthly visits for infants and children <5 years of age and two monthly for older children. Adequate dietetic time is required for both clinic contacts and telephone advice.[69]

5.28 Nutritional guidelines as shown in Table 2 should be followed for the child with CRF, and adjusted when dialysis commences.[69,71] If a child is within the normal percentile of ranges for height (>2nd percentile) then the energy requirements can be based upon the recommendations for children of the same chronological age. If the child falls below the normal percentile of ranges for height (<2nd percentile), the child's height age may be used to determine the acceptable baseline for energy requirements and adjusted accordingly thereafter.[71]

Table 2. Nutritional recommendations for children with CRF and on dialysis.

Age	Energy (per kg body wt/day)		Protein (per kg body wt/day)(g)		Phosphate (mg/day)
	cal	kj	pre-dialysis and HD	PD	
Infants					
Preterm	120–180	500–750	2.5–3.0	3.0–4.0	<400 mg (<10 kg body wt)
0–0.5 yr	115–150	480–630	1.5–2.1	2.1–3.0	<600 mg (10–20 kg body wt)
0.5–1.0	95–150	400–630	1.5–1.8	2.0–3.0	<800 mg (20–40 kg body wt)
1.0–2.0	95–120	400–500	1.0–1.8	2.0–3.0	<1000 mg (>40 kg body wt)
Children/ adolescents	Minimum of EAR for chronological				
2.0–puberty	age, or height		10.–1.5	1.5–2.0	
pubertal	age if <2nd		1.0–1.5	1.4–1.8	
post-pubertal	centile for height		1.0–1.5	1.3–1.5	

EAR = estimated average requirement, Dietary reference values, 1991.[71]
Protein intake should be at least the reference nutrient intake (RNI).[71]

5.29   Assessment of growth should be undertaken by staff who have received training in the use of appropriate measurement techniques and equipment. Supine length or standing height, weight and head circumference (in children under five years of age) should be plotted on reference growth charts for healthy children.[68] The weight and height velocity (and head circumference in young children) are reliable indicators of growth and probably the most sensitive indicators of nutritional progress. Height velocity must be calculated for the year before and then annually during rhGH therapy, and rhGH side effects must be audited. The current recommended dose of rhGH is 10 mg/m^2/week. When starting a child on rhGH, parental heights should be measured to ascertain the child's target height. Preliminary investigations should include fasting plasma glucose and insulin levels, thyroid function and bone age. Glucose and insulin levels should be repeated six monthly, along with a full anthropometric assessment. RhGH should be stopped if there is no improvement in growth, if there are side effects, or if the child receives a renal transplant. It should not be restarted within one year to allow time to ascertain whether post transplant catch-up growth will occur. Consideration may be given to stopping rhGH in all children when the growth velocity has fallen to the pre rhGH value or if the child has reached the centile for their target height. Any potential side effects must be reported.

Recommendation

▶ Many children with CRF have renal dysplasia with renal tubular losses of salt and water that may require salt supplementation. (C)

References

1   USRDS 1992 Annual Data Report. Comorbid conditions and correlations with mortality risk among 3,399 incident hemodialysis patients. *Am J Kidney Dis* 1992;**20**:32–8.

2   Owen WF, Lew NL, Liu Y *et al.* The urea reduction ratio and serum albumin concentration as predictors of mortality in patients undergoing hemodialysis. *N Engl J Med* 1993;**329**:1001–06.

3   Goldwasser P, Mittman N, Antignani A *et al.* Predictors of mortality in hemodialysis patients. *J Am Soc Nephrol* 1993;**3**:1613–22.

4   Foley RN, Parfrey PS, Harnett JD *et al.* Hypoalbuminemia, cardiac morbidity, and mortality in end-stage renal disease. *J Am Soc Nephrol* 1996;**7**:728–36.

5   Salem MM, Bower J. Hypertension in the hemodialysis population: any relation to one-year survival? *Am J Kidney Dis* 1996;**28**:737–40.

6   Iseki K, Miyasato F, Tokuyama K *et al.* Low diastolic blood pressure, hypoalbuminemia, and risk of death in a cohort of chronic hemodialysis patients. *Kidney Int* 1997;**51**:1212–17.

7   Jones CH, Newstead CG, Will EJ, Davison AM. Serum albumin and survival in CAPD patients: the implications of concentration trends over time. *Nephrol Dial Transplant* 1997;**12**:554–58.

8   Gamba G, Mejia JL, Saldivar S *et al.* Death risk in CAPD patients. The predictive value of the initial clinical and laboratory variables. *Nephron* 1993;**65**:23–7.

9   Churchill DN, Taylor DW, Cook RJ *et al.* Canadian Hemodialysis Morbidity Study. *Am J Kidney Dis* 1992;**19**:214–34.

10 Jones CH, Smye SW, Newstead CG *et al.* Extracellular fluid volume determined by bioelectrical impedance and serum albumin in CAPD patients. *Nephrol Dial Transplant* 1998;**13**:393–97.

11 Kaysen GA, Schoenfeld PY. Albumin homeostasis in patients undergoing continuous ambulatory peritoneal dialysis. *Kidney Int* 1984;**25**:107–14.

12 Kaysen GA, Rathore V, Shearer G, Depner TA. Mechanisms of hypoalbuminemia in hemodialysis patients. *Kidney Int* 1995;**48**:510–16.

13 Jones CH, Newstead CG, Will EJ *et al.* Assessment of nutritional status in CAPD patients: serum albumin is not a useful measure. *Nephrol Dial Transplant* 1997;**12**:1406–13.

14 Owen WF, Lowrie EG. C-reactive protein as an outcome predictor for maintenance hemodialysis patients. *Kidney Int* 1998;**54**:627–36.

15 Ikizler TA, Wingard RL, Harvell J *et al.* Association of morbidity with markers of nutrition and inflammation in chronic hemodialysis patients: A prospective study. *Kidney Int* 1999;**55**:1945–51.

16 Stenvinkel P, Heimburger O, Paultre F *et al.* Strong association between malnutrition, inflammation, and atherosclerosis in chronic renal failure. *Kidney Int* 1999;**55**:1899–1911.

17 Zimmermann J, Herrlinger S, Pruy A *et al.* Inflammation enhances cardiovascular risk and mortality in hemodialysis patients. *Kidney Int* 1999;**55**:648–58.

18 Yang CS, Chen SW, Chiang CH *et al.* Effects of increasing dialysis dose on serum albumin and mortality in hemodialysis patients. *Am J Kidney Dis* 1996;**27**.

19 Eustace JA, Coresh J, Kutchey C *et al.* Randomized double-blind trial of oral essential amino acids for dialysis-associated hypoalbuminaemia. *Kidney Int* 2000;**57**:2527–38.

20 Wells FE, Addison GM, Postlethwaite RJ. Albumin analysis in serum of haemodialysis patients: discrepancies between bromocresol purple, bromocresol green and electroimmunoassay. *Ann Clin Biochem* 1985;**22**:304–9.

21 Carfray A, Patel K, Whitaker P *et al*. Albumin as an outcome measure in haemodialysis in patients: the effect of variation in assay method. *Nephrol Dial Transplant* 2000;**15**:1819–22.

22 Ansell D, Feest T (eds). The UK Renal Registry. *The third annual report*, 2000: Bristol: UK Renal Registry, 2000.

23 Uribarri J. Mild metabolic acidosis and protein metabolism in dialysis patients: a reasoned approach to alkali therapy. *Semin Dial* 1999;**12**:278–81.

24 Miller AL. Plasma bicarbonate assays – time for a new look? *Ann Clin Biochem* 1993;**30**:233-7.

25 Lowrie EG, Lew NL. Commonly measured laboratory variables in hemodialysis patients: relationships among them and to death risk. *Semin Nephrol* 1992;**12**:276–83.

26 Stein A, Moorhouse J, Iles-Smith H *et al*. Role of an improvement in acid-base status and nutrition in CAPD. *Kidney Int* 1997;**52**:1089–95.

27 Tsuchihashi K, Takizawa H, Torii T *et al*. Hypoparathyroidism potentiates cardiovascular complications through disturbed calcium metabolism: possible risk of vitamin D(3) analog administration in dialysis patients with end-stage renal disease. *Nephron* 2000;**84**:13–20.

28 Metcalfe W, Khan IH, Prescott GJ *et al*. Can we improve early mortality in patients receiving renal replacement therapy? *Kidney Int* 2000;**57**:2539–45.

29 Brancaccio D, Gallieni M, Cozzolino M. Treatment of hyperparathyroidism – why is it crucial to control serum phosphate? [editorial]. *Nephrol Dial Transplant* 1996;**11**:420–3.

30 Nestico PF, DePace NL, Kotler MN *et al*. Calcium phosphorus metabolism in dialysis patients with and without mitral anular calcium. Analysis of 30 patients. *Am J Cardiol* 1983;**51**:497–500.

31 Forman MB, Virmani R, Robertson RM, Stone WJ. Mitral anular calcification in chronic renal failure. *Chest* 1984;**85**:367–71.

32 Maher ER, Young G, Smyth-Walsh B *et al*. Aortic and mitral valve calcification in patients with end-stage renal disease. *Lancet* 1987;**2**:875–7.

33 Huting J. Predictive value of mitral and aortic valve sclerosis for survival in end-stage renal disease on continuous ambulatory peritoneal dialysis. *Nephron* 1993;**64**:63–8.

34 Goldsmith DJ, Covic A, Sambrook PA, Ackrill P. Vascular calcification in long-term haemodialysis patients in a single unit: a retrospective analysis. *Nephron* 1997;**77**:37–43.

35 Altmann P, Al-Salihi F, Butter K *et al*. Serum aluminum levels and erythrocyte dihydropteridine reductase activity in patients on hemodialysis. *N Engl J Med* 1987;**317**:80–4.

36 Altmann P, Dhanesha U, Hamon C *et al*. Disturbance of cerebral function by aluminium in haemodialysis patients without overt aluminium toxicity [see comments]. *Lancet* 1989;**2**:7–12.

37 Iseki K, Uehara H, Nishime K *et al*. Impact of the initial levels of laboratory variables on survival in chronic dialysis patients. *Am J Kidney Dis* 1996;**28**:541–8.

38 Block GA, Hulbert-Shearon TE, Levin NW, Port FK. Association of serum phosphorus and calcium x phosphate product with mortality risk in chronic hemodialysis patients: a national study. *Am J Kidney Dis* 1998;**31**:607–17.

39 Chertow GM, Lowrie EG, Lew NL, Lazarus M. Mineral metabolism and mortality in haemodialysis (abstract). *J Am Soc Nephrol* 2000;**11**:560A.

40 Foley RN, Parfrey PS, Harnett JD *et al*. Hypocalcaemia, morbidity, and mortality in end-stage renal disease. *Am J Nephrol* 1996;**16**:386–93.

41 Anonymous. Diagnosis and treatment of aluminium overload in end-stage renal failure patients. *Nephrol Dial Transplant* 1993;**8**:1–4.

42 Degoulet P, Legrain M, Reach I *et al*. Mortality risk factors in patients treated by chronic hemodialysis. Report of the Diaphane collaborative study. *Nephron* 1982;**31**:103–10.

43 Lowrie EG, Lew NL. Death risk in hemodialysis patients: the predictive value of commonly measured variables and an evaluation of death rate differences between facilities. *Am J Kidney Dis* 1990;**15**:458–82.

44 De Lima JJG, Sesso R, Abensur H *et al*. Predictors of mortality in long-term haemodialysis patients with a low prevalence of comorbid conditions. *Nephrol Dial Transplant* 1995;**10**:1708–13.

45 Clinical practice guidelines for nutrition in chronic renal failure. K/DOQI, National Kidney Foundation. *Am J Kidney Dis* 2000;**35**:S1–140.

46 Malnutrition Advisory Group of the British Association for Parenteral and Enteral Nutrition. *Guidelines for the detection and management of malnutrition*. Maidenhead: BAPEN, 2000.

47 World Health Organization. *Physical status: the use and interpretation of anthropometry*. Geneva: WHO, 1995.

48 Windsor JA, Hill GL. Weight loss with physiologic impairment – a basic indicator of surgical risk. *Ann Surg* 1988;**207**:290–6.

49 Canada-USA (CANUSA) Peritoneal Dialysis Study Group. Adequacy of dialysis and nutrition in continuous peritoneal dialysis: association with clinical outcomes. *J Am Soc Nephrol* 1996;**7**: 198–207.

50 Detsky AS, McLaughlin JR, Baker JP *et al*. What is subjective global assessment of nutritional status? *JPEN J Parenter Enteral Nutr* 1987;**11**:8–13.

51 Ikizler TA, Greene JH, Wingard RL *et al*. Spontaneous dietary protein intake during progression of chronic renal failure. *J Am Soc Nephrol* 1995;**6**:1386–91.

52 Kopple JD, Greene T, Chumlea WC *et al*. Relationship between nutritional status and the glomerular filtration rate: results from the MDRD study. *Kidney Int* 2000;**57**:1688–703.

53 Kaysen GA. Malnutrition and the acute-phase reaction in dialysis patients-how to measure and how to distinguish. *Nephrol Dial Transplant* 2000;**15**:1521–4.

54 Stenvinkel P, Heimburger O, Lindholm B *et al*. Are there two types of malnutrition in chronic renal failure? Evidence for relationships between malnutrition, inflammation and atherosclerosis (MIA syndrome). *Nephrol Dial Transplant* 2000;**15**:953–60.

55 Louden JD, Roberts RR, Goodship TH. Acidosis and nutrition. *Kidney Int Suppl* 1999;**73**:S85–8.

56 Stratton RJ, Elia M. A critical systematic analysis of the use of oral nutritional supplements in the community. *Clin Nutr* 1998;**18** (Suppl 2):29–84.

57 Jones M, Hagen T, Boyle CA *et al*. Treatment of malnutrition with 1.1% amino acid peritoneal dialysis solution: results of a multicenter outpatient study. *Am J Kidney Dis* 1998;**32**:761–9.

58 Foulks CJ. An evidence-based evaluation of intradialytic parenteral nutrition. *Am J Kidney Dis* 1999;**33**:186–92.

59 Report of the Panel on Dietary Reference Values of the Committee on Medical Aspects of Food Policy. *Dietary reference values for food, energy and nutrients for the United Kingdom*. Vol. 41. London: HMSO, 1991;152–5.

60 Taubes G. The (political) science of salt. *Science* 1998;**281**:898–901, 903–7.

61 Greenland P. Beating high blood pressure with low-sodium DASH. *N Engl J Med* 2001;**344**:53–5.

62 Sacks FM, Svetkey LP, Vollmer WM *et al*. Effects on blood pressure of reduced dietary sodium and the Dietary Approaches to Stop Hypertension (DASH) diet. DASH-Sodium Collaborative Research Group. *N Engl J Med* 2001;**344**:3–10.

63 Krautzig S, Janssen U, Koch KM *et al*. Dietary salt restriction and reduction of dialysate sodium to control hypertension in maintenance haemodialysis patients. *Nephrol Dial Transplant* 1998;**13**:552–3.

64 World Health Organization. *Physical status: the use and interpretation of anthropometry*. Vol. 854. Geneva: WHO, 1995;312–44.

65 Kopple JD, Zhu X, Lew NL, Lowrie EG. Body weight-for-height relationships predict mortality in maintenance hemodialysis patients. *Kidney Int* 1999;**56**:1136–48.

66   Fleischmann EH, Bower JD, Salahudeen AK. Risk factor paradox in hemodialysis: better nutrition as a partial explanation. *ASAIO J* 2001;**47**:74–81.

67   Malluche HH, Ritz E, Lange HP *et al.* Bone histology in incipient and advanced renal failure. *Kidney Int* 1976;**9**:355–62.

68   Freeman JV, Cole TJ, Chinn S *et al.* Cross-sectional stature and weight reference curves for the UK. *Arch Dis Child* 1990;**73**:17–24.

69   Coleman JE. The kidney. In: Shaw V, Lawson M (eds). *Clinical paediatric dietetics.* Oxford: Blackwell Scientific Publications,1994;125–42.

70   Kari JA, Gonzalez C, Lederman SE *et al.* Outcome and growth of infants with severe chronic renal failure. *Kidney Int* 2000;**57**:1681–87.

71   Department of Health Report on Health and Social Subjects No 41. *Dietary reference values for food, energy and nutrients for the United Kingdom.* London: HMSO, 1991.

6 Cardiovascular risk factors in patients on dialysis

Introduction

6.1   Cardiovascular disease is a prominent cause of premature death in dialysis patients. The increased risk compared with the general population is more prominent in younger patients, such that a 35-year old haemodialysis (HD) patient has the same risk of death from cardiovascular disease as an 80-year old in the general population.[1]

6.2   Replacement of renal function by dialysis is an intermediate treatment for many patients with end stage renal disease (ESRD) who will ultimately be treated by transplantation. Very little evidence is available on whether treatments known to reduce cardiovascular risk in the general population are also effective in patients with ESRD, and there is a pressing need for clinical trials in this area. It is illogical, however, to assume that treatments known to be of benefit in one phase of chronic renal failure (CRF) will not continue to be beneficial when a patient enters a different phase. Thus a patient with hypercholesterolaemia, who receives evidence-based statin treatment early in the natural history of their illness, should not have this withdrawn when they begin HD (and total cholesterol falls). Nor, for example, should a patient with left ventricular hypertrophy (LVH) receiving a beta-blocker or angiotensin converting enzyme (ACE) inhibitor, have that therapy withdrawn when they commence HD.

6.3   It should be made clear that individual risk factors, such as blood pressure, should not be viewed in isolation. Hence, in a patient with essential hypertension and LVH, control of blood pressure without regression of LVH would be perceived as inadequate treatment. Similarly, non-renal patients with heart failure and low blood pressure still benefit from beta-blockade and ACE inhibition.

6.4   Interpretation of the observational data relating potential risk markers to outcomes in dialysis patients is confounded by reverse causation – in which the marker is affected by pre-existing disease.[2] For instance, heart failure caused by poorly controlled hypertension results in a fall in blood pressure, to the extent that low blood pressure identifies a group with a high risk of death.

Blood pressure

Standards

▶ Pre-haemodialysis systolic blood pressure should be below 140 mmHg. **(C)**

▶ Pre-haemodialysis diastolic blood pressure should be below 90 mmHg. **(C)**

▶ Post-dialysis systolic blood pressure should be below 130 mmHg. **(C)**

▶ Post-dialysis diastolic blood pressure should be below 80 mmHg. **(C)**

▶ Post-dialysis blood pressure should be recorded after completion of dialysis, including washback. **(Good practice)**

▶ Blood pressure in patients on peritoneal dialysis (PD) should be below 130 mmHg systolic and 80 mmHg diastolic. **(C)**

Recommendation

▶ Blood pressure should be measured according to the recommendations of the British Hypertension Society, in the non-fistula arm with an appropriate cuff size, with the patient seated comfortably for five minutes prior to measurement, following 30 minutes abstention from caffeine and nicotine. The arm should be supported at heart level and at least two measurements of blood pressure should be taken, either with a mercury sphygmomanometer or with a validated electronic device. A third should be taken if there is a significant discrepancy between the first two. The mean of the last two measurements should be recorded. **(Good practice)**

RATIONALE

6.5   Cardiovascular disease is the dominant cause of premature death amongst patients on renal replacement therapy (RRT), and therefore a major target for intervention. Hypertension is a feature of early renal disease, and its prevalence reaches 90% amongst patients nearing ESRD.[3] LVH is related both to hypertension[4–8] and possibly to anaemia,[4,8,9] although this association may be artefactual, due to overestimation of LV mass as a result of the cardiac dilatation which results from anaemia.[10] LVH is a powerful predictor of premature death amongst patients on dialysis.[11–14] Hypertension and ischaemic heart disease are both precursors of heart failure and left ventricular dilatation, which is an even more powerful predictor for early death in dialysis patients.[6] Hypertension may be difficult to control in dialysis patients despite multiple medications.[15] Hypertension which is refractory to combination antihypertensive medication is frequently due to subclinical salt and water overload, even in the absence of peripheral or pulmonary oedema.[16,17] Adequate control of extracellular volume by ultrafiltration is, therefore, the 'first line' treatment for hypertension in HD patients.

6.6   Several large recent studies have shown an association between low blood pressure and increased mortality in dialysis patients,[6,18–20] or have shown a U-shaped relationship, with both low and high blood pressure being associated with an increased relative risk of death.[21] It is likely that these more modern studies included a higher proportion of patients with established cardiac disease, and the most likely explanation for the findings is that cardiac failure, whether due to hypertensive heart disease or to ischaemic heart disease, carries a high risk of mortality and is associated with low blood pressure.

6.7   The weight of evidence points to hypertension, often sustained for many years longer than the observation periods of the studies cited above, as a major cause of cardiac damage and eventually of cardiac failure, low blood pressure, and death. A recent paper supports this interpretation: in a single centre study, early mortality was associated with low diastolic blood pressure, but late mortality was associated with high systolic blood pressure.[22] However, there have been no controlled trials examining the effect of blood pressure reduction on outcome in HD patients. Such trials would be complicated because blood pressure control can be achieved by both fluid removal and drug therapy in dialysis patients. One French centre[23,24] has shown excellent patient survival using slow fluid removal and salt restriction alone, but their results may have been confounded by patient selection.

Pre-dialysis or post-dialysis measurements?

6.8   Most studies of blood pressure in HD patients have used pre-dialysis blood pressure measurements on the assumption that these are more representative of blood pressure in the interdialytic period than measurements taken immediately after completion of dialysis, when the patient is still adapting to rapid reduction in extracellular volume (tending to cause hypotension) and to reduction in serum potassium (which causes vasoconstriction in skeletal muscle and hypertension).[25] However, several ambulatory blood pressure monitoring studies[26–8] have shown a closer relationship between mean ambulatory blood pressure and post-dialysis blood pressure than with pre-dialysis blood pressure, and post-dialysis measurements may be more predictive of outcome.[21]

Measurement of blood pressure

6.9   In the management of essential hypertension, the need for care in the interpretation of blood pressure measurements, and the unreliability of casual measurements, taken while the patient is stressed or anxious, are well recognised. Current recommendations suggest that blood pressure should be taken after five minutes rest in a chair, after at least 30 minutes of abstention from caffeine or nicotine, with the patient seated comfortably, and with the arm supported at heart level. At least two measurements should be taken, several minutes apart, to allow for the alerting response to blood pressure measurement (which is seen even in 'seasoned' patients). If the second measurement is significantly lower than the first, a third measurement should be taken, with further repeats if there is a further fall in measured blood pressure. The blood pressure recorded should be the mean of the later measurements.[29–32] There is no reason not to adopt similar standards for dialysis patients, and indeed it seems common sense to expect that casual, hurried measurements of blood pressure in a stressed patient just prior to the commencement of dialysis (involving needling of the fistula) may give misleadingly high readings.

6.10   Measurement of blood pressure may result in important changes in drug or dialysis prescription, and must therefore be reliable and accurate. With the forthcoming ban on the routine use of mercury sphygmomanometers, increasing reliance will be placed on semi-automatic devices. Standards for validation of these devices have been drawn up by the American Association of the Advancement of Medical Instrumentation (AAMI) and the British Hypertension Society (www.hyp.ac.uk/nhs/management/html); many devices in widespread use do not meet these standards.[33]

Age-related standards?

6.11   The previous edition of this document suggested a higher standard, 160/90 mmHg, for patients over 60 years of age than for younger patients (140/90 mmHg). In the general population, systolic hypertension is more common in the elderly, probably due to decreased large vessel compliance. Recent studies have shown that increased pulse pressure, a result of decreased conduit artery compliance,[34] is a much more powerful risk factor for death in the general population than systolic or diastolic blood pressure.[35–40] It has been shown recently that the absolute benefits of blood pressure reduction are greater in the elderly than in younger patients, due to the former having higher baseline risk, and that isolated systolic hypertension or combined systolic and diastolic hypertension in patients up to the age of 80 can be safely treated with good results.[41] However, many of the elderly patients in these trials had marked systolic hypertension, and the question of whether there is benefit from reducing systolic blood pressure from 160 mmHg to, say, 130 mmHg, has not been specifically examined in this patient group, or even in the general population. Setting a more liberal standard for blood pressure in the elderly risks giving the message that control of hypertension is less important in these patients, when the reverse is probably the case. For these reasons, the targets set here are independent of age.

Are the standards achievable?

6.12   There is a danger that if the standard set is widely seen as unrealistic, no effort will be made to achieve it. We know that blood pressure is substantially higher than these standards in many UK dialysis patients,[42,43] implying that a major change in practice will have to occur if the standards are to be reached. Some have argued that poor control of blood pressure is an inevitable result of shorter dialysis times, resulting in poorer control of salt and water balance and drug-resistant hypertension.[17] However, setting more liberal standards would risk allowing many more dialysis patients to develop clinical disease as a result of poor blood pressure control. Further research is urgently needed on blood pressure control strategies in dialysis patients. Continuing audit by the UK Renal Registry will show how many patients achieve the standards.

Identification and management of cardiac dysfunction

Recommendation

▶ All dialysis patients should have unimpeded access to echocardiography for the identification of LVH and LV dysfunction. (**Good practice**)

RATIONALE

6.13   Hypertension is associated with end-organ damage including renal damage and renal allograft dysfunction. In dialysis patients, the most apparent site of end-organ damage is the heart, where the vast majority of patients have evidence of LVH. This has a proven, adverse prognostic influence on patient outcome.[12–14] As in other patient groups, the control of blood pressure should be aimed at regression or prevention of end-organ damage.

6.14   Compared to the general population, one of the differences in the natural history of cardiovascular disease in dialysis patients is the relative infrequency of classical myocardial infarction and the over-representation of sudden, presumed arrhythmic deaths.[44,45] The increased mortality of patients with LVH and LV dysfunction can be explained by an increased risk of localised cardiac ischaemia and increased arrhythmogenicity. The use of beta-blockers reduces the risk of peri-operative myocardial infarction in high-risk patients[46–9] and is likely to have similar effects in high-risk dialysis patients. It has been argued that beta-blockers are under-used in high-risk dialysis patients, eg those with diabetes.[50] Beta-blockade should therefore be considered, irrespective of blood pressure, in dialysis patients with electrocardiogram (ECG) or echocardiographic abnormalities associated with increased risk of death.

Recommendations

▶ All dialysis units should record the development of left ventricular failure (see explanation in 6.15) in a manner permitting audit of the management of such patients. (**Good practice**)

▶ All patients with suspected heart failure should be investigated using echocardiography. (**Good practice**)

▶ All patients with proven systolic heart failure should receive treatment with ACE inhibitors and low-dose beta-blockers unless specifically contraindicated. (**B**)

RATIONALE

6.15   Circulatory congestion in patients with normal hearts can mimic the clinical signs of congestive cardiac failure.[51] There is therefore at least a theoretical difficulty in accurately distinguishing dialysis patients with heart failure from those with pure saline overload as a result of excessive ingestion of salt and water, inaccurate prescription of fluid removal on dialysis, or both. Treatments of known benefit for heart failure due to hypertension or ischaemic heart disease are unlikely to be of benefit in patients with pure fluid overload. The fact remains, however, that dialysis patients presenting with clinical symptoms and signs of heart failure, whatever the exact pathophysiology, have a very poor prognosis,[12,52–4] and it is likely that many such patients do in fact have heart disease, in view of the high prevalence of abnormal systolic function amongst dialysis patients.[14] Certainly, it should not be assumed that pulmonary oedema in a dialysis patient results from fluid overload alone, and patients presenting with pulmonary oedema should be investigated to exclude acute or recent myocardial infarction and to examine systolic function using echocardiography. It is possible that the causes of abnormal systolic function in dialysis patients are different from those in the general population with heart failure; however, hypertension and ischaemic heart disease are probably the most important contributors. Control of the symptoms of heart failure by ultrafiltration alone may therefore be equivalent to management of heart failure in the non-renal patient by diuretics alone, a strategy associated with increased neurohormonal activation and a poor outcome.

6.16   Prescription of ACE inhibitors to non-renal patients with systolic heart failure has important prognostic benefits,[55–7] as does the prescription of slowly increasing doses of beta-blockers.[55,57,58] Both classes of drug are widely used in dialysis patients, and there is no reason to expect that the prognostic advantage they confer in heart failure would not also be seen in patients on dialysis.

6.17   Spironolactone has also been shown to be of benefit in severe heart failure,[59] but there is less certainty that these advantages would also be seen in dialysis patients. Many clinicians would be concerned that spironolactone might interfere with extra-renal disposal of a potassium load, either by affecting translocation into cells or colonic secretion, although the evidence that spironolactone has these effects in anephric patients is limited.[60] Digoxin is of symptomatic benefit in heart failure, but its use requires careful dose adjustment in renal failure.

| **Recommendations** |

▶ Smoking habits should be recorded in dialysis patients in a manner permitting audit and should be actively discouraged in all those with a reasonable life expectancy and strongly discouraged in those on the transplant waiting list. (**Good practice**)

▶ Exercise should be encouraged. (**Good practice**)

▶ Glycosylated haemoglobin (HbA1c) should be below 7% in dialysis patients with diabetes, measured using an assay method which has been harmonised to the Diabetes Control and Complications Trial (DCCT) standard. (**B**)

▶ 3 hydroxy-3 methylglutaryl-Co-enzyme A (HMG–CoA) reductase inhibitors should be considered for primary prevention in dialysis patients with a 10-year risk of coronary disease, calculated as ≥30% according to the Joint British Societies' chart or the coronary risk calculator, ignoring the fact that these calculations may not be accurate in patients with renal disease. A total cholesterol of <5 mmol/l or a 30% reduction from baseline, or a fasting low density lipoprotein (LDL)-cholesterol of <3 mmol/l, should be achieved, whichever is the greatest reduction. (**C**)

▶ HMG–CoA reductase inhibitors should not be withdrawn from patients in whom they were previously indicated and prescribed when such patients start renal replacement therapy (RRT) or change modality. (**C**)

▶ Serum or red cell folate should be above the lower limit of the reference range in patients on dialysis. (**Good practice**)

RATIONALE

6.18   Cigarette smoking is associated with an increased cardiovascular risk in the general population, with more rapid progression of CRF[61–3] and with cardiovascular mortality following transplantation.[64,65]

6.19   Exercise is of proven benefit in reducing cardiovascular risk in the general population, acting via a number of mechanisms including the promotion of negative energy balance resulting in weight loss.[32] Although exercise tolerance may be limited in dialysis patients by anaemia and by abnormal muscle metabolism, there is no reason to believe that the benefits seen in the general population would not also apply to dialysis patients.

6.20   Cardiovascular mortality is higher in diabetic patients on dialysis than in non-diabetics.[66,67] This finding is extrapolated from those applying to the general population.[32] There is no evidence specific to renal failure which demonstrates a benefit from tight diabetes control, although a retrospective analysis of diabetic patients starting PD showed poorer survival in those whose diabetes had been poorly controlled in the six months prior to initiation of dialysis.[68]

6.21   Hyperlipidaemia is common in dialysis patients; the pattern is an elevated triglyceride value, low high density lipoprotein (HDL)-cholesterol, variable changes in LDL and total cholesterol. All are dependent on nutrition, co-morbidity and dialysis modality. There are no studies of the effect of lipid-lowering interventions on outcome in this population. Large-scale epidemiological studies in HD patients have shown an inverse or U-shaped relationship between serum cholesterol and subsequent mortality.[69-73] This inverse association is probably a good example of reverse causation: chronic disease, chronic inflammation, and malnutrition all cause hypocholesterolaemia and are independent risk markers for death. There is no reason to suppose that hyper-cholesterolaemia does not have the same role in atherogenesis as it does in patients without renal disease. Two studies in continuous ambulatory peritoneal dialysis (CAPD) patients have shown a direct correlation between total cholesterol or total:HDL-cholesterol ratio and survival.[74,75] Evidence linking triglyceride levels to outcome in dialysis patients is even less certain than it is in the general population. Several ongoing studies, including UK-HARP and Die Deutsche Diabetes Dialyse (4D), will inform this debate.

6.22   Treatment designed to lower cardiovascular risk is only cost-effective if targeted at patients who are at high risk of atherosclerotic events. This is the principle behind the Joint British Societies' Guidelines, in which a risk table or coronary risk calculator (available at http://www.hyp.ac.uk/bhs/risk.xls) is used to estimate risk.

6.23   Treatment with HMG–CoA reductase inhibitors ('statins') has been shown to be highly effective at reducing the risk of atherosclerotic events in patients at risk for such events, the degree of protection being higher, the greater the initial risk. Although the major action of this class of drugs is the reduction of total serum cholesterol concentration, there may be other potentially beneficial actions including anti-oxidant and immunomodulatory effects. Estimation of cardiovascular risk will require accurate recording of data for each dialysis patient regarding smoking, family history of premature vascular disease, blood pressure, total and HDL-cholesterol, and the presence or absence of diabetes, in addition to age and sex.

6.24   In case-control studies, plasma homocysteine levels are frequently higher in patients with clinical evidence of vascular disease than in those without, both in the general population and in renal disease; hyperhomocysteinaemia is common even in minor renal impairment.[76] Correction of folic acid deficiency, if present, reduces plasma homocysteine levels in patients with renal impairment but even very high doses (eg 60 mg daily) of folic acid or methylated derivates do not completely normalise homocysteine levels. The evidence that hyperhomocysteinaemia is causally related to atherogenesis from longitudinal studies is less persuasive than that from cross-sectional studies.[77] There is as yet very little evidence that intervention to lower homocysteine levels affects the risk of disease, either in the general population or in renal disease. However, correction of folate deficiency is good clinical practice irrespective of any possible effect on homocysteine levels or vascular disease risk.

Recommendations

▶ All dialysis units should record myocardial infarction, stroke, transient ischaemic attacks, and symptomatic peripheral vascular disease events in a manner permitting audit of the management of such patients. (**Good practice**)

▶ All dialysis patients with a history of myocardial infarction, stroke, peripheral vascular disease, acute coronary syndrome, or who undergo surgical or angiographic coronary revascularisation should be treated with aspirin, an ACE inhibitor, a beta-blocker, and an HMG–CoA reductase inhibitor unless contraindicated. Doses of ACE inhibitors and beta-blockers should be the maximum tolerated. (**C**)

▶ In patients in whom lipid-lowering drug treatment is used, total cholesterol should be reduced by 30% or to below 5 mmol/l, or LDL-cholesterol to below 3 mmol/l, whichever reduction is the greatest. (**C**)

▶ Dialysis patients should have unimpeded access to a full range of cardiac investigations including exercise echocardiography, radio-isotopic cardiac scans, and coronary angiography. (**Good practice**)

RATIONALE

6.25 Survival after myocardial infarction in dialysis patients is very poor.[78,79] Most of the informative large studies have included few patients with renal disease or have specifically excluded such patients. There is no reason, however, to expect that the important survival advantages conferred by treatment with ACE inhibitors, beta-adrenergic blockers, and HMG–CoA reductase inhibitors would not apply to patients with renal disease. Guidelines for the management of non-renal patients with proven ischaemic heart disease should be followed.[32]

6.26 Diagnosis of coronary disease in dialysis patients may be problematic. Angina with normal coronary arteries is not uncommon,[80,81] but is matched by an equally high prevalence of clinically silent coronary disease.[82] Standard exercise electrocardiography is unreliable as a result of poor exercise tolerance and a high prevalence of pre-existing electrocardiographic abnormalities. Minimising premature deaths by revascularisation in patients with prognostically important coronary disease requires accurate identification of such patients; many will only be identified by coronary angiography. It is particularly important to identify patients on the waiting list for transplantation who might have coronary disease, to minimise the risk of intra- or post-operative death from myocardial infarction either by removing such patients from the list or by revascularisation. Risk markers for the presence of coronary artery disease in dialysis patients include:

▶ symptomatic angina

▶ unexplained arrythmias

▶ recurrent dialysis-related hypotension

▶ heart failure, ECG abnormalities, and

▶ wall motion abnormalities on echocardiography.

6.27 There are no randomised controlled trials available comparing modern medical management with percutaneous or surgical revascularisation in patients with renal disease. It is reasonable to expect that the prognostic significance of, for example, triple vessel disease compared to single vessel disease is similar in renal patients and in the general population, and that the benefits of revascularisation on prognosis in high risk patients are similar. However, observational data point to a high rate of re-stenosis after angioplasty in dialysis patients and to an increased risk of complications after surgical evascularisation. Decisions on whether a patient is 'fit' for renal transplantation, therefore, have to be made on an individual basis. These decisions will also be influenced by local policy governing access to the transplant waiting list (see Chapter 8).

Other interventions in secondary prevention

6.28 Several non-enzymatic modifications of LDL particles enhance their uptake by scavenger receptors and increase the atherogenicity of LDL. These include oxidation, carbamylation, and the formation of advanced glycation end products. Patients with renal disease have decreased antioxidant defence. One recent small placebo-controlled randomised controlled trial (RCT) of vitamin E (800 IU/day, in dialysis patients with established vascular disease), showed a remarkable decrease in further events.[83] These results are in contrast to much larger studies in the general population. Pending confirmation of the beneficial effects of vitamin E in renal failure, no firm recommendations can be made on the routine prescription of antioxidants as primary or secondary preventive treatment in dialysis patients.

Paediatric section

6.29 Children with CRF will have a lifetime of treatment ahead of them and therefore it is important to focus on those aspects of management that may decrease the risks of cardiovascular disease. There is evidence that even young children have signs of early atherosclerosis.[84] The role of lipid lowering is controversial,[85] so the single most important area for prevention of cardiovascular disease is, at present, control of the blood pressure. Although children do not typically suffer overt hypertensive disease, there is accumulating evidence that systolic blood pressure elevation is as important a factor in the morbidity of hypertension in children as it is in adults.[86]

Blood pressure

Standard

▶ Blood pressure varies throughout childhood and should be maintained within two standard deviations of the mean for normal children of the same height and sex.[87] (C)

Recommendations

▶ The systolic blood pressure during pre-terminal CRF should be maintained at <90th centile for age, gender and height. (C)

▶ The systolic blood pressure during PD should be maintained at <90th centile for age, gender and height. Parents should be taught blood pressure recording and provided with appropriate equipment for measurement at home. (C)

▶ The systolic blood pressure after HD should be maintained at <90th centile for age, gender and height. In those with sustained hypertension, parents should be taught blood pressure recording and be provided with appropriate equipment for measurement on the days between dialyses, as this may be more representative of overall control than pre-dialysis blood pressure. **(C)**

▶ 'Whitecoat' hypertension does occur in children and is compounded by the pressure effect of the automated blood pressure devices. Twenty-four hour ambulatory blood pressure monitoring in children should be available in all tertiary paediatric centres.[88] **(Good practice)**

▶ Echocardiography in hypertensive patients is recommended at yearly intervals as a minimum. **(Good practice)**

Lipids

Recommendations

▶ Fasting cholesterol and trigylceride levels should be measured in all children commencing renal replacement therapy and at annual intervals. **(Good practice)**

▶ The dietetic advice from the paediatric renal dietitian for children over two years of age should take into consideration nutritional guidelines on cardiovascular disease and the document *The balance of good health*.[88–91] **(C)**

References

1 Parfrey PS, Foley RN. The clinical epidemiology of cardiac disease in chronic renal failure. *J Am Soc Nephrol* 1999;**10**:1606–15.

2 Baigent C, Burbury K, Wheeler D. Premature cardiovascular disease in chronic renal failure. *Lancet* 2000;**356**:147–52.

3 Buckalew VM Jr, Berg RL *et al*. Prevalence of hypertension in 1,795 subjects with chronic renal disease: the modification of diet in renal disease study baseline cohort. Modification of Diet in Renal Disease Study Group. *Am J Kidney Dis* 1996;**28**:811–21.

4 Levin A, Singer J, Thompson CR *et al*. Prevalent left ventricular hypertrophy in the predialysis population: identifying opportunities for intervention. *Am J Kidney Dis* 1996;**27**:347–54.

5 Harnett JD, Kent GM, Barre PE *et al*. Risk factors for the development of left ventricular hypertrophy in a prospectively followed cohort of dialysis patients. *J Am Soc Nephrol* 1994;**4**:1486–90.

6 Foley RN, Parfrey PS, Harnett JD *et al*. Impact of hypertension on cardiomyopathy, morbidity, and mortality in end-stage renal disease. *Kidney Int* 1996;**49**:1379–85.

7 Savage T, Giles M, Tomson CV, Raine AEG. Gender differences in mediators of left ventricular hypertrophy in dialysis patients. *Clin Nephrol* 1998;**49**:107–12.

8 Tucker B, Fabbian F, Giles M *et al*. Left ventricular hypertrophy and ambulatory blood pressure monitoring in chronic renal failure. *Nephrol Dial Transplant* 1997;**12**:724–8.

9 Silberberg JS, Rahal DP, Patton DR, Sniderman AD. Role of anemia in the pathogenesis of left ventricular hypertrophy in end-stage renal disease. *Am J Cardiol* 1989;**64**:222–4.

10 Stewart GA, Foster J, Cowan M *et al*. Echocardiography overestimates left ventricular mass in hemodialysis patients relative to magnetic resonance imaging. *Kidney Int* 1999;**56**:2248–53.

11 Silberberg JS, Barre PE, Prichard SS, Sniderman AD. Impact of left ventricular hypertrophy on survival in end-stage renal disease. *Kidney Int* 1989;**36**:286–90.

12 Parfrey PS, Griffiths SM, Harnett JD *et al*. Outcome of congestive heart failure, dilated cardiomyopathy, hypertrophic hyperkinetic disease, and ischemic heart disease in dialysis patients. *Am J Nephrol* 1990;**10**:213–21.

13 Foley RN, Parfrey PS, Hanrett JD *et al*. Clinical and echocardiographic disease in patients starting end-stage renal disease therapy. *Kidney Int* 1995;**47**:186–92.

14 Foley RN, Parfrey PS, Harnett JD *et al*. The prognostic signficance of left ventricular geometry in uremic cardiomyopathy. *J Am Soc Nephrol* 1995;**5**:2024–31.

15 Rahman M, Dixit A, Donley V *et al*. Factors associated with inadequate blood pressure control in hypertensive hemodialysis patients. *Am J Kidney Dis* 1999;**33**:498–506.

16 Fishbane S, Natke E, Maesaka JK. Role of volume overload in dialysis-refractory hypertension. *Am J Kidney Dis* 1996;**28**:257–61.

17 Scribner BH. Can antihypertensive medications control BP in haemodialysis patients: yes or no? *Nephrol Dial Transplant* 1999;**14**:2599–601.

18 USRDS 1992 Annual Data Report. Comorbid conditions and correlations with mortality risk among 3,399 incident hemodialysis patients. *Am J Kidney Dis* 1992;**20**:32–8.

19 Iseki K, Miyasato F, Tokuyama K *et al*. Low diastolic blood pressure, hypoalbuminemia, and risk of death in a cohort of chronic hemodialysis patients. *Kidney Int* 1997;**51**:1212–17.

20 Port FK, Hulbert-Shearon TE, Wolfe RA *et al*. Predialysis blood pressure and mortality risk in a national sample of maintenance hemodialysis patients. *Am J Kidney Dis* 1999;**33**:507–17.

21 Zager PG, Nikolic J, Brown RH *et al*. 'U' curve association of blood pressure and mortality in hemodialysis patients. Medical Directors of Dialysis Clinic, Inc [erratum in *Kidney Int* 1998 Oct;54(4): 1417.] *Kidney Int* 1998;**54**:561–9.

22 Mazzuchi N, Carbonell E, Fernandez-Cean J. Importance of blood pressure control in hemodialysis patient survival. *Kidney Int* 2000;**58**:2147–54.

23 Charra B, Calemard E, Ruffet M *et al*. Survival as an index of the adequacy of dialysis. *Kidney Int* 1992;**41**.

24 Charra B, Calemard E, Laurent G. Importance of treatment time and blood pressure control in achieving long-term survival on dialysis. *Am J Nephrol* 1997;**16**:35–44.

25 Dolson GM, Adrogue HJ. Low dialysate [K+] decreases efficiency of hemodialysis and increases urea rebound. *J Am Soc Nephrol* 1998;**9**:2124–28.

26 Kooman JP, Gladziwa U, Bocker G *et al*. Blood pressure during the in terdialytic period in haemodialysis patients: estimation of representative blood pressure values. *Nephrol Dial Transplant* 1992;**7**:917–23.

27 Coomer RW, Schulman G, Breyer JA, Shyr Y. Ambulatory blood pressure monitoring in dialysis patients and estimation of mean interdialytic blood pressure. *Am J Kidney Dis* 1997;**29**:678–84.

28 Mitra S, Chandna SM, Farrington K. What is hypertension in chronic haemodialysis? The role of interdialytic blood pressure monitoring. *Nephrol Dial Transplant* 1999; **14**:2915–21.

29 Ramsay L, Williams B, Johnston G *et al*. Guidelines for management of hypertension: report of the third working party of the British Hypertension Society. *J Hum Hypertens* 1999;**13**:569–92.

30 1999 World Health Organization–International Society of Hypertension Guidelines for the Management of Hypertension. Guidelines Subcommittee. *J Hypertens* 1999;**17**:151–83.

31 The sixth report of the Joint National Committee on prevention, detection, evaluation, and treatment of high blood pressure [erratum in *Arch Intern Med* 1998 Mar 23;**158**(6):573]. *Arch Intern Med* 1997;**157**:2413–46.

32 Joint British recommendations on prevention of coronary heart disease in clinical practice. British Cardiac Society, British Hyperlipidaemia Association, British Hypertension Society, endorsed by the British Diabetic Association. *Heart* 1998;**80**(Suppl 2):S1–29.

33 O'Brien E, Waeber B, Parati G *et al*. Blood pressure measuring devices: recommendations of the European Society of Hypertension. *BMJ* 2001;**322**:531–6.

34 Blacher J, Guerin AP, Pannier B *et al*. Impact of aortic stiffness on survival in end-stage renal disease. *Circulation* 1999;**99**:2434–9.

35   Benetos A, Safar M, Rudnichi A *et al*. Pulse pressure: a predictor of long-term cardiovascular mortality in a French male population. *Hypertension* 1997;**30**:1410–15.

36   Benetos A, Rudnichi A, Safar M, Guize L. Pulse pressure and cardiovascular mortality in normotensive and hypertensive subjects. *Hypertension* 1998;**32**:560–4.

37   Mitchell GF, Moye LA, Braunwald E *et al*. Sphygmomanometrically determined pulse pressure is a powerful independent predictor of recurrent events after myocardial infarction in patients with impaired left ventricular function. SAVE investigators. Survival and Ventricular Enlargement. *Circulation* 1997;**96**:4254–60.

38   Franklin SS, Khan SA, Wong ND *et al*. Is pulse pressure useful in predicting risk for coronary heart Disease? The Framingham heart study. *Circulation* 1999;**100**:354–60.

39   Millar JA, Lever AF, Burke V. Pulse pressure as a risk factor for cardiovascular events in the MRC Mild Hypertension Trial. *J Hypertens* 1999;**17**:1065–72.

40   Glynn RJ, Chae CU, Guralnik JM *et al*. Pulse pressure and mortality in older people. *Arch Intern Med* 2000;**160**:2765–72.

41   Lever AF, Ramsay LE. Treatment of hypertension in the elderly. *J Hypertens* 1995;**13**:571–9.

42   Ansell D, Feest T (eds). The UK Renal Registry: *The second annual report*, 1999: Bristol: UK Renal Registry, 1999.

43   Ansell D, Feest T (eds). The UK Renal Registry: *The third annual report*, 2000: Bristol: UK Renal Registry, 2000.

44   Parfrey PS, Foley RN, Harnett JD *et al*. Outcome and risk factors of ischemic heart disease in chronic uremia. *Kidney Int* 1996;**49**:1428–34.

45   Chazan JA, Pono LM. Sudden death in patients with chronic renal failure on hemodialysis. *Dial Transplant* 1987;**16**:447–8.

46   Mangano DT, Layug EL, Wallace A, Tateo I. Effect of atenolol on mortality and cardiovascular morbidity after noncardiac surgery. Multicenter Study of Perioperative Ischemia Research Group. *N Engl J Med* 1996;**335**:1713–20.

47   Eagle KA, Froehlich JB. Reducing cardiovascular risk in patients undergoing noncardiac surgery. *N Engl J Med* 1996;**335**:1761–3.

48   Poldermans D, Boersma E, Bax JJ *et al*. The effect of bisoprolol on perioperative mortality and myocardial infarction in high-risk patients undergoing vascular surgery. Dutch Echocardiographic Cardiac Risk Evaluation Applying Stress Echocardiography Study Group. *N Engl J Med* 1999;**341**:1789–94.

49   Lee TH. Reducing cardiac risk in noncardiac surgery. *N Engl J Med* 1999;**341**:1838–40.

50   Zuanetti G, Maggioni AP, Keane W, Ritz E. Nephrologists neglect administration of betablockers to dialysed diabetic patients. *Nephrol Dial Transplant* 1997;**12**:2497–500.

51   Eichna LW. Non-cardiac circulatory congestion simulating congestive cardiac failure. *Trans Assoc Am Physicians* 1954;**67**:72–83.

52   Hutchinson TA, Thomas DC, MacGibbon B. Predicting survival in adults with end-stage renal disease: an age equivalence index. *Ann Intern Med* 1982;**96**:417–23.

53   Harnett JD, Foley RN, Kent GM *et al*. Congestive heart failure in dialysis patients: prevalence, incidence, prognosis and risk factors. *Kidney Int* 1995;**47**:884–90.

54   Foley RN, Parfrey PS, Harnett JD *et al*. Hypoalbuminemia, cardiac morbidity, and mortality in end-stage renal disease. *J Am Soc Nephrol* 1996;**7**:728–36.

55   The treatment of heart failure. Task Force of the Working Group on Heart Failure of the European Society of Cardiology. *Eur Heart J* 1997;**18**:736–53.

56   Flather MD, Yusuf S, Kober L *et al*. Long-term ACE-inhibitor therapy in patients with heart failure or left-ventricular dysfunction: a systematic overview of data from individual patients. ACE-Inhibitor Myocardial Infarction Collaborative Group. *Lancet* 2000;**355**:1575–81.

57   Consensus recommendations for the management of chronic heart failure. On behalf of the membership of the advisory council to improve outcomes nationwide in heart failure. *Am J Cardiol* 1999;**83**:1A–38A.

58   Krumholz HM. b-blockers for mild to moderate heart failure. *Lancet* 1999;**353**:2–3.

59   Pitt B, Zannad F, Remme WJ *et al*. The effect of spironolactone on morbidity and mortality in patients with severe heart failure. Randomized Aldactone Evaluation Study Investigators. *N Engl J Med* 1999;**341**:709–17.

60   Sugarman A, Brown RS. The role of aldosterone in potassium tolerance: studies in anephric humans. *Kidney Int* 1988;**34**:397–403.

61   Bleyer AJ, Shemanski LR, Burke GL *et al*. Tobacco, hypertension, and vascular disease: risk factors for renal functional decline in an older population. *Kidney Int* 2000;**57**:2072–9.

62   Halimi JM, Giraudeau B, Vol S et al. Effects of current smoking and smoking discontinuation on renal function and proteinuria in the general population. *Kidney Int* 2000;**58**:1285–92.

63   Stengel B, Couchoud C, Cenee S, Hemon D. Age, blood pressure and smoking effects on chronic renal failure in primary glomerular nephropathies. *Kidney Int* 2000;**57**:2519–26.

64   Cosio FG, Falkenhain ME, Pesavento TE *et al*. Patient survival after renal transplantation: II. The impact of smoking. *Clin Transplant* 1999;**13**:336–41.

65   Kasiske BL, Klinger D. Cigarette smoking in renal transplant recipients. *J Am Soc Nephrol* 2000;**11**:753–9.

66   Ritz E, Strumpf C, Katz F *et al*. Hypertension and cardiovascular risk factors in hemodialyzed diabetic patients. *Hypertension* 1985;**7**:II118–24.

67   Ritz E, lippert J, Keller C. Hypertension, cardiovascular complications and survival in diabetic patients on maintenance haemodialysis. *Nephrol Dial Transplant* 1995;**10**(Suppl 7):43–6.

68   Wu MS, Yu CC, Yang CW *et al*. Poor pre-dialysis glycaemic control is a predictor of mortality in type II diabetic patients on maintenance haemodialysis. *Nephrol Dial Transplant* 1997;**12**:2105–10.

69   Pollock CA, Ibels LS, Caterson RJ *et al*. Continuous ambulatory peritoneal dialysis. Eight years of experience at a single center. *Medicine* 1989;**68**:293–308.

70   Lowrie EG, Lew NL. Death risk in hemodialysis patients: the predictive value of commonly measured variables and an evaluation of death rate differences between facilities. *Am J Kidney Dis* 1990;**15**:458–82.

71   Lowrie EG, Lew NL. Commonly measured laboratory variables in hemodialysis patients: relationships among them and to death risk. *Semin Nephrol* 1992;**12**:276–83.

72   Goldwasser P, Mittman N, Antignani A *et al*. Predictors of mortality in hemodialysis patients. *J Am Soc Nephrol* 1993;**3**:1613–22.

73   Piccoli GB, Quarello F, Salomone M *et al*. Are serum albumin and cholesterol reliable outcome markers in elderly dialysis patients? *Nephrol Dial Transplant* 1995;**10**:72–7.

74   Gamba G, Mejia JL, Saldivar S *et al*. Death risk in CAPD patients. The predictive value of the initial clinical and laboratory variables. *Nephron* 1993;**65**:23–7.

75   Little J, Phillips L, Russell L *et al*. Longitudinal lipid profiles on CAPD: their relationship to weight gain, comorbidity, and dialysis factors. *J Am Soc Nephrol* 1998;**9**:1931–9.

76   Bostom AG, Culleton BF. Hyperhomocysteinemia in chronic renal disease. *J Am Soc Nephrol* 1999;**10**:891–900.

77   Christen WG, Ajani UA, Glynn RJ, Hennekens CH. Blood levels of homocysteine and increased risks of cardiovascular disease: causal or casual? *Arch Intern Med* 2000;**160**:422–34.

78   Chertow GM, Normand SL, Silva LR, McNeil BJ. Survival after acute myocardial infarction in patients with end-stage renal disease: results from the cooperative cardiovascular project [see comments]. *Am J Kidney Dis* 2000;**35**:1044–51.

79   Herzog CA. Poor long-term survival of dialysis patients after acute myocardial infarction: bad treatment or bad disease? [editorial; comment]. *Am J Kidney Dis* 2000;**35**:1217–20.

80   Roig E, Betriu A, Castaner A *et al*. Disabling angina pectoris with normal coronary arteries in patients undergoing long-term hemodialysis. *Am J Med* 1981;**71**:431–4.

81   Rostand SG, Kirk KA, Rutsky EA. Dialysis-associated ischemic heart disease: insights from coronary angiography. *Kidney Int* 1984;**25**:653–9.

82   Kremastinos D, Paraskevaidis I, Voudiklari S *et al*. Painless myocardial ischemia in chronic hemodialysed patients: a real event? *Nephron* 1992;**60**:164–70.

83   Boaz M, Smetana S, Weinstein T *et al*. Secondary prevention with antioxidants of cardiovascular disease in endstage renal disease (SPACE): randomised placebo-controlled trial. *Lancet* 2000;**356**:1213–18.

84   Kari JA, Donald AE, Vallance DT *et al*. Physiology and biochemistry of endothelial function in children with chronic renal failure. *Kidney Int* 1997;**52**:468–472.

85   Querfeld U. Should hyperlipidaemia in children with the nephrotic syndrome be treated? *Pediatr Nephrol* 1999;**13**:77–84.

86   Sorof JM. Systolic hypertension in children – benign or beware? *Pediatr Nephrol* 2001;**16**:517–25.

87   The Update on the 1987 Task Force Report on High Blood Pressure in Children and Adolescents: A Working Group Report from the National High Blood Pressure Education Program. *Pediatr* 1996;**98**:649–58.

88   Soergel M, Kirshstein M, Busch C *et al*. Oscillometric twenty-four-hour ambulatory blood pressure values in healthy children and adolescents: a multicenter trial including 1141 subjects. *J Pediatr* 1997;**130**:178–84.

89   Coleman JE. The kidney. In: Shaw V, Lawson M (eds). *Clinical paediatric dietetics*, 2nd edn. Boston: Blackwell Science, 2001;158–82.

90   Department of Health. Committee on Medical Aspects of Food Policy. Nutritional Aspects of Cardiovascular Disease. *Reports on health and social subjects 46*. London: HMSO, 1994.

91   Health Education Authority. *The balance of good health*. London: HEA, 1996.

7 Anaemia in patients with chronic renal failure

Adult section

7.1 The anaemia of chronic renal failure (CRF) is of particular importance because of its major impact on patient morbidity and perhaps mortality, and the high per patient cost of correction. Up to 2000, fifty-nine randomised controlled trials (RCTs) were identified in the area of anaemia in renal failure and six questions have been addressed, some of them in systematic reviews. Nevertheless many areas remain uncertain and are the subject of current studies, particularly on whether haemoglobin should be normalised and how epoetin should be used before dialysis is required. The evidence base for recommendations therefore varies in strength. The recommendations here apply to patients for whom dialysis is not yet required and to those already established on treatment.

Standards

▶ Target haemoglobin: patients with CRF should achieve a haemoglobin of 10 g/dl **(A)*** within six months of being seen by a nephrologist, unless there is a specific reason such as those outlined below. It is unclear as yet how epoetin should be used optimally in patients before dialysis becomes necessary and whether normalisation of haemoglobin gives further benefit.

▶ Adequate iron status. Patients must be iron replete to achieve and maintain target haemoglobin whether receiving epoetin or not. **(B)** A definition of adequate iron status is a serum ferritin >100 µg/l and <10% hypochromic red cells (transferrin saturation >20%).**

Recommendations

▶ Evaluate anaemia in CRF when Hb<12 g/dl (adult males and post-menopausal females), <11 g/dl (pre-menopausal females) **(B)**; anaemia may be considered the result of uraemia if the glomerular filtration rate (GFR) is <30 ml/min (<45 ml/min in diabetics) and no other cause, eg blood loss, folate or B12 deficiency, is identified. **(B)**

▶ Iron administration: oral iron will in general be sufficient to attain and maintain the above targets in those not yet requiring dialysis and those on peritoneal dialysis (PD); in contrast, many haemodialysis (HD) patients will require intravenous iron. **(B)**

▶ Regular monitoring of iron status (at least every six months) is essential during treatment to avoid toxicity: a serum ferritin consistently greater than 800 µg/l is suggestive of iron overload. **(B)**

continued

---

* Level A evidence so far only for dialysis patients.
** Pre-dialysis blood sample in those on haemodialysis.

▶ Route of epoetin administration: it is preferable to give epoetin subcutaneously even in HD patients. **(A)** Some patients (such as obese subjects) may require intravenous injection to obtain good absorption.

▶ Haemoglobin concentration should be monitored monthly for stable hospital HD patients and 3–4 monthly for stable home HD and PD patients and epoetin dosage adjusted accordingly. **(C)** Haemoglobin will require more frequent monitoring to begin with.

▶ 'Resistance' to epoetin: failure to reach the target, or need for doses of epoetin above 300 IU/kg/week, defines inadequate response ('resistance'). Iron deficiency (absolute or functional) remains the commonest cause. Hyporesponsive patients who are iron replete should be screened clinically and by laboratory testing for other common causes, such as raised immunoreactive parathyroid hormone (iPTH), malignancy, infection/inflammation, aluminium toxicity, effect of angiotensin converting enzyme (ACE) inhibitors and possibly epoetin antibodies. **(B)**

▶ Blood pressure: must be monitored in all patients receiving epoetin, and hypertension if present (for definition see Chapter 6) should be treated by volume removal and/or hypotensive drugs. **(B)**

7.2   Many renal units, particularly large ones, find it helpful to use computer algorithms to maximise their ability to achieve the target haemoglobin for as many patients as possible. For 85% of the population to achieve a haemoglobin of ≥10 g/dl the population median requires to be 11.5 g/dl with current practice.[1] (Population target median for ferritin is 200–500 ug/l and for hypochromic red cells <2.5% (transferrin saturation (TSAT) 30–40%)).

RATIONALE

7.3   The anaemia of any patient with CRF should be corrected firstly by optimising dialysis and nutrition (including an adequate supply of iron); and secondly by correction of epoetin deficiency if, despite these measures, the haemoglobin remains below the target concentration. Epoetin therapy, however, must not be used as a support for inadequate dialysis.[2] There are likely to be opportunities for savings as well as costs in the use of epoetin, arising from the prevention of later complications, especially those requiring expensive investigations and/or hospital admission. There are, however, few data available on the cost effectiveness of this treatment.

7.4   There is abundant evidence from prospective randomised controlled trials of patients on dialysis that shows that during epoetin treatment, there are improvements in:

▶   quality of life

▶   exercise capacity

▶   cardiac function

▶   sleep patterns

▶   cognitive functioning

▶   immune responses, and

▶   sexual function.

Medicare data from the USA suggest that hospital admission rates and total expenditure per patient may be less for those on epoetin.[3] Although no prospective randomised controlled study has yet shown an improvement in patient survival with a rise in haemoglobin, one uncontrolled prospective study[4] and a number of retrospective studies[5] suggest that survival is better in such patients. Such studies may be confounded because the factors causing the anaemia rather than the anaemia itself may lead to the unfavourable outcome.

7.5   It appears also that in uraemic patients who do not yet require dialysis, anaemia is an important predictor of cardiac morbidity and mortality, with their attendant costs.[6] Investigation and management of anaemia should begin before dialysis is required. How epoetin should be used optimally to treat this patient group is the subject of current investigation and, hence, for the present, we suggest the same target haemoglobin for this group. Despite some suggestions from animal models that improvement in anaemia accelerates the rate of decline in renal function, current evidence does not allow any firm conclusions to be drawn on whether or not this applies to humans.[7] One uncontrolled study in the USA indicated improved survival in patients given epoetin before dialysis became necessary, but patients in this group were also more likely to have had health insurance before dialysis, be in employment, and have started dialysis electively.[8]

7.6   The haemoglobin concentration that should be aimed for ('target haemoglobin') remains controversial. Because of the high cost of epoetin treatment, the minimum amount of haemoglobin and epoetin necessary to improve measurable functions was sought, rather than aiming for correction to normal concentrations. Current evidence from RCTs of dialysis patients supports only a correction to between 9.5 and 11g/dl.[9–10] The former large trial[9] included only patients with cardiovascular disease and was not completed because of the higher death rate in the group where an attempt was made to normalise haemoglobin. There were many problems, however, with the data obtained.[11] Considerable evidence from as yet unpublished RCTs and smaller cohort studies with short follow-up, suggest that further improvements in physical and psychological functions may be obtained with normalisation of haemoglobin in some patient groups.[12–15] It may therefore be that, in the future, haemoglobin targets should be tailored to the individual rather than aiming for a single target haemoglobin for all patients in a dialysis unit. A proportion of patients, particularly those on PD and those not yet requiring dialysis, may not need epoetin to attain the target above, particularly if well nourished, iron replete and well dialysed.

7.7   Although the European Best Practice Guidelines[16] suggest a higher target haemoglobin (11 g/dl), for the moment we prefer to keep the concentration recommended in the two previous editions of this document. What will prove to be the most cost-effective concentration of haemoglobin should emerge in the near future, and will be kept under review. Fears of increased access thrombosis and vascular disease following normalisation of haemoglobin[9] have not been confirmed in further uncontrolled (or as yet unpublished) studies of patients either with[15,17] or without[13] vascular disease. Blood pressure must be monitored but hypertension is controllable with increased ultrafiltration and/or hypotensive agents.

7.8   There is good evidence that the use of concomitant iron both improves attained haemoglobin concentration and reduces doses of epoetin required to reach target haemoglobin.[16] The two should be regarded as synergistic in the treatment of the anaemia of renal failure, and epoetin should not be given without iron supplementation. In general, in patients not yet on dialysis and those on PD, it is useful to begin using oral iron, even though this is poorly absorbed and tolerated in renal failure. The effect of concomitant treatments (eg phosphate binders) on iron absorption must be taken into account. In patients on HD, however, because of greater continuing iron losses from the dialysis procedure and blood sampling, intravenous iron may be necessary.[16] Two large RCTs draw opposite conclusions on whether intravenous iron should be used routinely[18–19] since although ferritin concentrations failed to improve during oral iron therapy in either trial, haemoglobin concentrations were equal for up to 24 weeks in the latter study. Intravenous iron is much more expensive than oral iron, but in HD patients final costs were similar from savings on epoetin dosage in another study.[20] No particular preparations or dosage regimens can be recommended over others at present. Iron dextran may cause allergic reactions and it is better to use other preparations which are as effective and do not carry this risk.

7.9   Iron deficiency can be recognised only by indirect tests at the moment and the limitations of the serum ferritin concentration, TSAT and even percentage of hypochromic erythrocyte measurements should be recognised. In particular, some patients who have apparently normal iron stores but fail to respond to epoetin adequately, may respond if further iron is given, usually by the intravenous route ('functional iron deficiency'). Careful monitoring is necessary to eliminate inadequate treatment but iron overload will also need to be avoided. At present many renal units do not have access to what has emerged as preferable indices of iron status, such as percentage of circulating hypochromic cells or the reticulocyte haemoglobin concentration.[21] Renal units should endeavour to bring these into use in collaboration with their colleagues in haematology.

7.10   Epoetin should be given subcutaneously in the first instance, since the dosage of maintenance epoetin required to produce equivalent responses are, in a meta-analysis of controlled trials, 40 IU/kg/week less with the subcutaneous than with the intravenous route.[22] A proportion of patients (eg those with gross obesity) will however require a lower dosage using the iv route.

7.11   A proportion of patients (15–20% of all those treated) fail to respond adequately with the expected rise in haemoglobin concentration within six months, and require higher doses than anticipated. An evidence-based definition of hypo-responsiveness ('resistance') to epoetin is failure to respond to >300 IU/kg/week (95th centile). Such patients require investigation (and if possible treatment) for haemoglobinopathies, iron deficiency, malignancies, inflammatory diseases, hyperparathyroidism, aluminium intoxication and a number of rarer conditions, as well as effects of drugs such as ACE inhibitors. A European Union directive and the American Food and Drug Administration have noted that resistance leading on to pure red cell aplasia has been reported in about 1:10,000 of patients treated mainly, but not exclusively, with epoetin alpha.[23] In such patients epoetin should be stopped, and anti-epoetin antibodies sought. Further advice on usage of epoetin alpha is awaited.

7.12   New types of erythropoiesis-stimulating agents are currently under trial, but there are too few data as yet to recommend what place they may have in the treatment of renal anaemia in the future. In particular, a more highly glycosylated substance with erythropoetic activity is now available, novel erythropoeisis stimulating protein (NESP),[24] or darbepoetin which has a much longer half-life after injection than conventional epoetin, and gene-activated epoetin delta. The long duration of action of darbepoetin could confer advantage in patients not on dialysis or on continuous ambulatory peritoneal dialysis (CAPD) as longer intervals between injections are possible.

7.13   Note: these recommendations were constructed in the light of detailed information summarised and evaluated in the *European best practice guidelines for the management of anaemia in patients with chronic renal failure*[16] to which the reader is referred for most of the supporting evidence underlying the above. The reader is also referred to the American Dialysis Outcomes Quality Initiative (DOQI) *Clinical practice guidelines for the treatment of anemia of chronic renal failure.*[25] Additional data published in 1998–2000, some of it cited above, have been evaluated and taken into account.

Paediatric section

7.14   Anaemia in children with CRF has additional importance as it may adversely affect appetite and growth. Correction of anaemia improves nutritional intake and is associated with improvement in growth, although this has not been shown in a controlled trial.[26]

Standards

▶ Target haemoglobin: all children with CRF and on dialysis should achieve their target haemoglobin within six months of seeing a paediatric nephrologist, unless there is a specific reason otherwise. Targets are age specific, as below:

▷ Children under six months of age should achieve a haemoglobin of greater than or equal to 9.5 g/dl.

▷ Children aged six months to two years should achieve a haemoglobin of greater than or equal to 10.0 g/dl.

▷ Children over two years of age should achieve a haemoglobin of greater than or equal to 10.5 g/dl. (**B**)

▶ Adequate iron status: all children should achieve a serum ferritin of greater than 100 µg/l and less than 800 µg/l, whether or not they are receiving epoetin. (**B**)

Recommendations

▶ Evaluation of anaemia: the haemoglobin rises throughout childhood as follows: normal range (±2 SD) before six months of age is 11.5 (9.5–13.5) g/dl; from six months to two years it is 12.0 (10.5–13.5) g/dl; and it rises progressively to 13.5 (11.5–15.5) g/dl by 12 years. Evaluate for anaemia when the haemoglobin falls to <10 g/dl before six months of age, <11 g/dl from six months to two years, and <12 g/dl in older children. (**Good practice**)

▶ Iron administration: persistently low ferritin despite oral supplementation is an indication for intravenous iron therapy. Side effects must be monitored. (**B**)

▶ Haemoglobin concentration should be monitored every 1–2 months. (**Good practice**)

▶ Iron status should be monitored every three months. (**Good practice**)

7.15   Epoetin is effective in children in improving the anaemia of CRF and dialysis, and in children with failing renal transplants.[26] Epoetin doses in children are comparable on a unit/kg basis to adult requirements[27] and have been shown to be safe. Subcutaneous injection is the most bioavailable route of administration. Dosage intervals can be determined by response, but are usually once to twice weekly.[28] Iron and folic acid supplementation is required.

References

1   Ansell D, Feest T (eds). The UK Renal Registry. *The second annual report*, 1999. Bristol: UK Renal Registry, 1999.

2   Ifudu O, Feldman J, Friedman EA. The intensity of hemodialysis and the response to erythropoietin in patients with end stage renal disease. *N Engl J Med* 1996;**334**:420-25.

3   Collins AJ, Li S, Ebben J *et al*. Hematocrit levels and associated Medicare expenditure. *Am J Kidney Dis* 2000;**36**:282–93.

4   Locatelli F, Conte F, Marcelli O. The impact of hematocrit levels and erythropoietin treatment on overall and cardiovascular mortality and morbidity – the experience of the Lombardy Dialysis Registry. *Nephrol Dial Transplant* 1998;**13**:1642–4.

5   Collins AJ, Ma J, Xia A, Ebben J. Trends in anemia treatment with erythropoietin usage and patient outcomes. *Am J Kidney Dis* 1998;**32**(suppl 4):S133–S41.

6   Levin A, Thompson CR, Ethier J *et al*. Left ventricular mass index increase in early renal disease: impact of decline in hemoglobin. *Am J Kidney Dis* 1999;**34**:125–34.

7   Cody J, Daly C, Campbell M *et al*. Systematic review of pre-dialysis erythropoietin use: an example of industry-funding of independent health technology. Edinburgh: International Society of Health Technology Assessment Congress, June 1999 (abstract).

8   Fink J, Blahut S, Reddy M, Light P. Use of erythropoietin before the initiation of dialysis and its impact on mortality. *Am J Kidney Dis* 2001;**37**(2):348–55.

9   Besarab A, Bolton WK, Browne JK *et al*. The effects of normal as compared with low hematocrit values in patients with cardiac disease who are receiving hemodialysis and epoetin. *N Engl J Med* 1998;**339**:584–90. [RCT]

10   Canadian Erythropoietin Study Group. Association between recombinant human erythropoietin and quality of life and exercise capacity of patients receiving haemodialysis. *Br Med J* 1990;**300**:573–8. [RCT]

11   Macdougall I (on behalf of the UK multicentre IV iron study group). UK multi-centre randomized controlled study of IV vs oral iron supplementation in dialysis patients receiving epoetin. *J Am Soc Nephrol* 1999;**10**:291A (abstract). [RCT]

12   McMahon LP, McKenna MJ, Sangkabutra T *et al*. Physical performance and associated electrolyte changes after haemoglobin normalization: a comparative study in haemodialysis patients. *Nephrol Dial Transplant* 1999;**14**:1182–7. [RCT]

13   Moreno F, Sanz-Guajardo D, Manuel J *et al*. Increasing hematocrit has a beneficial effect on Quality of Life and is safe in selected hemodialysis patients. *J Am Soc Nephrol* 2000:**101**:335–42.

14   Picket JL, Theberge DC, Brown WS *et al*. Normalizing hematocrit in dialysis patients improves brain function. *Am J Kidney Dis* 1999;**33**:1122–30.

15   Scandinavian erythropoietin study: effects on quality of life of normalizing hemoglobin levels in uremic patients. *J Am Soc Nephrol* 1999;**10**:269A (abstract). [RCT]

16 Working Party for European Best Practice Guidelines. European Best Practice Guidelines for the management of anaemia in patients with chronic renal failure. *Nephrol Dial Transplant* 2000;**15**, Suppl 4.

17 European Study on Anaemia Management (ESAM). Unpublished data presented at the XXXIVth meeting of the European Renal Association, Madrid, 5th September 1999.

18 Fishbane S, Frei GL, Masaeka J. Reduction in recombinant erythropoietin doses by the use of chronic intravenous iron supplementation. *Am J Kidney Dis* 1995;**26**:41–6. [RCT]

19 Macdougall IC, Ritz E. The normal hematocrit trial in dialysis patients with cardiac disease: are we any less confused about target haemoglobin? *Nephrol Dial Transplant* 1998;**13**:3030–3.

20 Stevens PE, Jenkins K, Swift PA *et al*. True costs of correction of anaemia in the dialysis population. *Nephrol Dial Transplant* 1999;**14**:A252.

21 Fishbane S, Shapiro W, Dutka P *et al*. A randomised trial of iron deficiency testing strategies in haemodialysis patients. *Kidney Int* 2001;**6**:2406–11.

22 Daly C, Pennington S, Cody J *et al*. Is intravenous administration of erythropoietin a waste of resources? *Nephrol Dial Transplant* 1999;**14**:A256 (abstract). [Systematic review]

23 Casadevell N, Nataf J, Viron B *et al*. Pure red cell aplasia and antierythropoietin antibodies in patients treated with recombinant erythropoietin. *N Engl J Med* 2002;**346**:469–75.

24 Locatelli F, Olivares J, Walker R *et al* on behalf of the European/Australian NESP 980202 study group. Novel erythropoiesis stimulating protein for treatment of anemia in chronic renal insufficiency. *Kidney Int* 2001;**60**:741–7.

25 National Kidney Foundation DOQI. *Clinical practice guidelines for the treatment of anaemia of chronic renal failure* (2nd version). New York: National Kidney Foundation, 2001.

26 Jabs K. The effects of recombinant human erythropoietin on growth and nutritional status. *Pediatr Nephrol* 1996;**10**:324–7.

27 Brandt JR. Safety and efficacy of erythropoietin in children with chronic renal failure. *Pediatr Nephrol* 1999;**13**:143–7.

28 Van Damme-Lombaerts R, Herman J. Erythropoietin treatment in children with renal failure. *Pediatr Nephrol* 1999;**13**:148–52.

8 | Transplantation

Introduction

8.1   Transplantation of a kidney, from either a living related or cadaver donor, can, if successful, give patients a life free of dialysis and all its attendant restrictions. The management of patients before, during and after transplantation is a multidisciplinary activity. This chapter has, therefore, been written in conjunction with the British Transplantation Society.

Access to transplantation and allocation of kidneys

Standard

▶ There must be demonstrable equity of access to donor organs irrespective of gender, race or district of residence. Age, of itself, is not a contra-indication to transplantation but age-related morbidity is important. **(Good practice)**

▶ All transplant units should have written criteria for acceptance on to the waiting list for renal transplantation, and all patients on dialysis should be offered the opportunity of assessment by nephrologists, transplant surgeons and transplant coordinators who should explain whether or not they are suitable for transplantation. The risks associated with transplantation should be fully explained verbally and in writing. **(Good practice)**

▶ All dialysis patients should have their suitability for transplantation reviewed at least annually, and recorded. Patients should be placed on or removed from transplant waiting lists only after discussion and agreement with nephrologists, transplant surgeons and the patients themselves. **(Good practice)**

▶ Kidneys should be allocated according to nationally agreed guidelines that take account of matching, waiting time, sensitisation and other factors. **(Good practice)**

RATIONALE

8.2   Renal transplantation remains the most successful and cost effective treatment for suitable patients with end stage renal disease (ESRD). The supply of cadaveric donor kidneys, which averaged 24 per million population per year in the UK in 1999 and 2000 (United Kingdom Transplant (UKT) data), is greatly outstripped by demand. For example, in the year 2000, 83 patients per million population were on the cadaveric transplant waiting list in the UK (UKT data). Cadaveric donor organs are thus an extremely valuable resource that must be used optimally. It is important also, however, that equity of access to transplantation is achieved.

8.3   Not all patients receiving dialysis are suitable for kidney transplantation and there is evidence[1] that selection criteria vary widely throughout the UK. This is reflected by the variation in the proportion of dialysis patients who are on the transplant waiting list in different regions. In addition, in some areas patients not yet on dialysis are accepted for cadaveric renal transplantation, and compete for organs with patients who may have been on dialysis for many years. Where there is a suitable live donor this form of 'pre-emptive transplantation' should be encouraged as it has a good outcome.[2]

8.4   In the UK definitive criteria for acceptance on to the cadaveric transplant waiting list have yet to be agreed although diabetes, vascular disease and a history of malignant disease are major co-morbid factors that reduce the likelihood of acceptance in many units. This attitude is based on poor survival of such recipients leading to premature death with a functioning graft. Practice guidelines regarding suitability for transplantation have been available in the USA for some years[3] and the European Best Practice Guidelines were published in 2000.[4]

8.5   In order to recommend standards for assessment of potential transplant recipients, further research on the significance of pre-transplant co-morbidity with respect to post-transplant outcome is required. This applies particularly to cardiovascular disease. In the meantime, individual transplant units should have written criteria regarding their acceptance of patients for renal transplantation, and all dialysis patients should have the opportunity to be assessed for renal transplantation and to be reassessed in another transplant unit if they disagree with their rejection after an initial assessment. At the time of assessment patients should be fully informed about the various risks of transplantation including surgical complications, drug side-effects, infection and malignant disease, both verbally and in writing.

8.6   Older age at the time of transplantation has generally been shown not to adversely affect short-term graft survival,[5,6] although age does have a major influence on longer-term patient survival.[7] However, the higher post-transplant mortality among older patients must be considered along with increasing evidence of a survival advantage of renal transplantation over dialysis at all ages.[8,9] At present only 6% of UK renal transplant recipients are over 65 years of age.

8.7   In 1998 a national allocation scheme for adult cadaveric kidneys was agreed by the UKT meeting. This scheme allocates kidneys on the basis of matching, and for equally matched recipients there is a points system which favours younger patients, those who have waited longer, those with rarer human major histocompatibility complex (HLA) types, those with lower sensitisation HLA antigens, those centres with a more positive balance of exchange, and transplants where there is closer age matching between recipients and donors. Since its introduction in July 1998 13% of kidneys have been given to 000 mismatched recipients, 48% to other favourably matched recipients (see 8.30), and the remainder to less well matched recipients (UKT data). This scheme is under annual review by the UKT users group.

8.8   The national allocation scheme needs further refinement to improve the equity of access for patients with unusual tissue types and less common blood groups as they are currently disadvantaged. Efforts to increase the organ donor rate from the ethnic minorities are ongoing and will also help to alleviate the above situation as patients from the ethnic minorities are more likely to fall into one of these categories. Recently a change to the allocation scheme has been made to help HLA homozygous recipients who were also disadvantaged in the original scheme.

▶ Services for kidney retrieval must be an integral part of organ transplant services and costed into them. (**Good practice**)

▶ Purchasers should fund efforts to increase the number of cadaver organs made available by the setting up of transplant coordination and organ procurement teams, and they should ensure that adequate educational programmes are in place; an important part of this is improved communication with intensive care units. (**Good practice**)

▶ An increase in live donor transplantation should be actively encouraged and living donors should remain under life-long follow-up. (**Good practice**)

RATIONALE

8.9   The kidney donation rate in the UK is twelfth among the 15 European Union (EU) countries and is therefore exceeded consistently by most Western European countries. The topic has been discussed extensively in a British Transplantation Society working party report which is, in turn, discussed by Wight and Cohen[10] as well as by the King's Fund.[11] Many topics remain unresolved. For example, standards for organs to be retrieved, methods for organ preservation and the use of non-heart-beating donors.

8.10   Educational activity regarding all aspects of organ donation should be developed throughout the UK, using transplant coordinators, and should be backed by adequate finance. Currently these services are inadequate and under-funded[12] and the costs associated with their expansion and improvement together with their formal recognition need to be met. Liaison with and involvement of intensivists and their staff is crucial.

8.11   The cost of organ retrieval needs to be included when costing renal services and taken into consideration by purchasers when constructing future budgets for transplantation of kidneys and other organs. Coordinator programmes are currently under review and may be supervised on a national basis by UKT in the future. UKT has recently appointed a Director of Communications, part of whose role will be to develop educational activity and material in conjunction with transplant coordinators.

8.12   Expansion of live donor transplantation has considerable potential for increasing the organ donation rate in the UK. In Norway, 18 live donor transplants are performed per million population per year. This compares with a figure of 5.7 per million population per year in the UK in 2000. The outcome of both live related and unrelated renal transplantation has been reported to be superior to that with cadaveric transplantation,[13] and the outlook for living kidney donors themselves is good.[14] A living organ donation programme requires great care to ensure that donation is altruistic, without coercion or reward, that the risks to the donor are minimised and that the requirements of the Human Organ Transplant Act 1989 are met in all respects. Guidelines for living donor kidney transplantation have been recently published by the British Transplantation Society.[15]

8.13   Living donors should be followed up to facilitate the collection of data on long-term morbidity and mortality. Information should be submitted for inclusion in the UK Live

Donor Register. Life-long follow-up is recommended.[15] The psychological response to donation is often positive. However, some donors may have significant psychological difficulties, particularly if the transplant has been unsuccessful and in such circumstances appropriate support should be available.

8.14 Simultaneous kidney and pancreas transplantation is not widely available to patients with ESRD secondary to Type 1 diabetes in the UK. A small number of UK transplant centres now offer this form of treatment, and if their results are similar to those reported by the International Pancreas Transplant Registry[16] then this form of transplantation should be made available to suitable recipients nationally.

The transplant unit

Recommendations

▶ Transplant units should, in general, serve at least two million total population, depending on geography, communications and population density. They should be appropriately located and preferably perform at least 50 transplants per year. (**Good practice**)

▶ Transplant units must be adequately staffed, both medically and surgically at senior and junior level, and have full support services, including a pathologist trained in the interpretation of renal transplant biopsies. Specialist advisory committee recommendations and junior doctors' hours guidelines must be followed. (**Good practice**)

▶ The care of the renal transplant recipient is best carried out by a multidisciplinary team with equal input from nephrologists and transplant surgeons. This element of care, along with full integration with the dialysis service, is essential. (**Good practice**)

RATIONALE

8.15 Renal transplantation facilities should be suitably located, taking into account geography, population density and communications. This avoids duplication of specialised resources such as histocompatibility laboratories and organ retrieval teams, and permits efficient training of medical and other staff.

8.16 The transplant unit should have four beds per million population available for new transplants, one third of which should be single-bed cubicles. This figure may need to be varied in the light of geography, communication networks and population density. The beds, with the facilities to provide dialysis when needed, must be within a single ward to ensure high standards of training, nursing and cross-infection care, although all the beds in the ward need not be devoted to transplantation.

8.17 Access to operating theatres 24 hours a day without delay to minimise the cold ischaemic time is essential[17] and, in addition, elective operating theatre facilities are needed. Laboratory support is required for histocompatibility and HLA antibody testing, haematology, biochemistry, virology, bacteriology and pathology. Histopathological services should include a pathologist trained in the interpretation of renal transplant biopsies. Imaging services required include routine X-ray, angiography, conventional and duplex ultrasound, computed tomography, magnetic resonance imaging and radioisotope scanning. It is important to emphasise that these services will often be required at short notice and out of normal working hours. Access to urology services and advice is necessary, and joint management of diabetic patients with a diabetologist is desirable before and after transplantation. For post-transplant surveillance, close links with cardiology, dermatology and gynaecology will be needed, and speedy access to other specialties such as neurology, gastroenterology, thoracic medicine and infectious disease will be required occasionally.

8.18   Patients should be followed up in a transplant clinic with appropriately trained and experienced staff. Consultant-led clinics will be needed for this although junior staff should participate under supervision, as may nurse practitioners. Recipients should be reviewed at least annually at a transplant centre unless the facilities in the devolved renal unit include the ability to transfer data centrally. In addition to monitoring and optimising renal function, follow-up clinics should consider cardiovascular risk management including:

▶   hypertension

▶   smoking

▶   diet

▶   exercise and dyslipidaemia

▶   prevention and detection of skin malignancy

▶   osteoporosis

▶   malignancy

▶   post-transplantation pregnancy and other women's health issues.

Blood pressure

Standard

▶ Blood pressure targets for renal transplant recipients are <130 mmHg systolic and <80 mmHg diastolic. **(B)**

8.19   Controlled trials of different blood pressure targets in renal transplant recipients are not available. In the meantime it is recommended that blood pressure control should have the same targets as in other patients with renal disease (see Chapter 10). Treatment of hyperlipidaemia and other preventive measures, including aspirin to prevent heart disease in diabetics, are recommended.[18,19] Controlled trials of the treatment of hypercholesterolaemia in renal transplant recipients are ongoing and, therefore, no firm recommendation for primary prevention can be made.[20,21] Prevention of osteoporosis should be aimed for by cessation of smoking, minimising corticosteroid exposure, encouraging exercise, hormone replacement therapy and adequate dietary calcium intake. Treatment of symptomatic osteoporosis should follow established guidelines.[22] Following graft failure, steroid therapy should be carefully withdrawn[23] and other immunosuppression stopped[24] whether or not the transplant kidney is removed.

8.20   Data storage and access for both clinical and service audit are essential: both staff and equipment must be costed into the service. The database should be interfaced with the UKT, which is integrated with the national Renal Registry. If patients are referred back for continuing care to local nephrologists, the local databases should be linked to the transplant unit.

8.21 Surgical staffing has been dealt with in detail in the review of renal services in England.[25] There should be at least four consultant surgeons trained in transplantation per two million population plus appropriate support staff; consultant rotas should not be more than one in four.[26] Cross cover by surgeons untrained in transplantation is not acceptable.

8.22 Multi-organ donation continues to increase and organ retrieval services must be designed with this in mind. Occasionally, recipients will receive kidney/liver and kidney/heart transplants. The services for these patients must be sited and administered with care, and joint management in transplant centres performing multiple transplants is desirable.

Histocompatibility matching and allocation of donor kidneys

Standards

▶ Sensitised recipients must have the HLA-specificities of circulating antibodies defined carefully. The sensitisation status of every patient registered on the national waiting list should be reviewed on at least an annual basis. **(B)**

▶ All donor recipient pairs should be cross-matched by an appropriate technique before transplantation. Flow cytometric cross-matching may be helpful for re-transplants and highly sensitised recipients. **(B)**

Recommendations

▶ An accredited tissue typing service is an essential part of a successful kidney transplant programme. Day-to-day direction of the laboratory must be provided by a medical or scientific consultant trained in histocompatibility and immunogenetics (H&I). The tissue typing laboratory staff must be an integral part of the transplant team. Laboratory staff must be available 24 hours a day to type and cross-match against donors. Living donors and recipients must be tested, as required under the terms of the Human Organ Transplants Act 1989. **(Good practice)**

▶ All centres should document local allocation criteria. Patient registration on the national waiting list must contain sufficient HLA typing and sensitisation information to support the operation of the allocation scheme. **(Good practice)**

▶ All screening for HLA-specific antibodies should use a typed panel that allows interpretation of positive reactions. The tissue-typing laboratory must be provided with patients' serum following sensitising events such as the transfusion of blood products or transplantation. Following transplantation, it is essential that the tissue-typing laboratory continues regularly to receive serum samples for antibody screening. Failure to provide these samples may jeopardise a patient's future chances of transplantation. All potential recipients must be screened regularly for HLA-specific antibodies. This should be at least every three months. **(Good practice)**

RATIONALE

8.23 Crucial to the provision of a quality service and the introduction of new developments are the staffing structure and personnel qualifications within the histocompatibility and immunogenetics (H&I) laboratory. The laboratory must be directed by a medical consultant, or a substantive consultant scientist (grade C clinical scientist) who is in charge of the day-to-day laboratory activity and is available for contact outside normal working hours. The director of the laboratory must have experience of working in an H&I laboratory and must have Membership of the Royal College of Pathologists in H&I, or evidence of at least an equivalent level of training in the subject.

8.24 Other scientific/technical staff should have successfully completed a recognised training scheme in H&I (British Society for Histocompatibility and Immunogenetics (BSHI) or Council for Professions Supplementary to Medicine (CPSM)), and should participate in relevant continuing professional development schemes. Trainees must participate in a recognised training scheme. It is, therefore, essential that training opportunities are provided within the laboratory for all personnel. The laboratory must be accredited by Clinical Pathology Accreditation (UK) Ltd (CPA), must participate in the UK National External Quality Assurance scheme (UK NEQAS) for each of the services offered and demonstrate an acceptable standard of performance.

8.25 It is important that close liaison is maintained between the laboratory and the clinical team. The head of the laboratory and other appropriate laboratory staff must therefore establish good professional relationships with the medical and professional staff in the transplant unit. Laboratory representation at relevant clinical and audit meetings is essential.

8.26 Technical developments in laboratory aspects of kidney transplantation have progressed rapidly and this is likely to continue. The advent of molecular biological techniques has had a significant impact on the quality of HLA typing and serological analysis. The introduction and use of novel cross-matching techniques has allowed the safe transplantation of otherwise high-risk transplant recipients. H&I laboratories will offer different repertoires of tests depending on the service(s) they provide and the transplant programme(s) they support. Descriptions of the tests that can be offered are given in the document, 'Standard tests in Histocompatibility & Immunogenetics', which can be obtained from the laboratory or from the BSHI. Each laboratory should provide a description of the tests offered and their clinical application.

8.27 The Human Organ Transplants (Establishment of Relationship) Regulations 1998 incorporated in the Human Organ Transplants Act 1989 state that for living donor transplantation, the genetic relationship between the proposed donor and recipient is to be established by means of genetic tests based on DNA variations. The tests are to be specified and the results interpreted by an 'approved tester' appointed by the Department of Health (DH). Where there is no claimed genetic relationship, or when such a relationship cannot be established, the case must be referred to the Unrelated Live Transplant Regulatory Authority (ULTRA) via the ULTRA Secretariat at the DH.

8.28 Approved testers must be fully aware of their responsibilities under the regulations, including receipt of signed statements claiming a relationship, documented blood samples, completion of specified tests, recording and long-term storage of test results and formal reporting. Testers must be aware of the limitations of the specified tests and should report accordingly. The penalties defined in the Act should be understood.

8.29 Identity or compatibility of ABO blood groups between donor and recipient currently is essential. The principle of matching the donor HLA type to that of the recipient to optimise transplant outcome and minimise rejection is well established and has been practised by UK units since 1970. Matching is especially important in determining longer term (5–15 years) outcomes.[27,28] As a minimum, for solid organ transplantation, all prospective donors and recipients must be typed for HLA-A, -B, -Cw, -DR, -DQ at the level required for the organ allocation programme.

8.30 In the UK, during 1997 and early 1998, the UK Transplant Users' Kidney Advisory Group developed and presented revised protocols for the allocation of kidneys based on a 3-tier system. The system for exchange of kidneys based on HLA matching and other factors affecting outcome is currently operated on the UK transplant community's behalf through UKT. In the allocation scheme, local patients have priority over other equally matched patients and certain groups of centres have formed waiting list alliances for organ allocation. The number of donor kidneys that are exported to other units and those received from elsewhere are recorded for each participating unit and openly monitored. All UK units are strongly encouraged to join the national scheme and register their potential recipients. The registration of patients must contain sufficient HLA typing and sensitisation information to support the operation of the national allocation scheme.

Favourable matching

8.31 A favourable match is defined as having a maximum of one mismatched antigen at either the HLA-A and HLA-B locus or at both (denoted 100, 010, 110). Recent analysis of UK data has shown significantly increased transplant survival in recipients of a 000 mismatched transplant. Also, favourably matched transplants had a significantly increased transplant survival when compared to transplants of other match grades.[17] 000 mismatched kidneys are allocated through tier 1; other favourably matched kidneys are allocated through tier 2. A points score is used as a discriminator should there be equally matched patients, currently based on recipient age, donor-recipient age difference, accumulated waiting time, sensitisation to HLA antigens, HLA antigen matchability and transplant unit balance of exchange. Wherever possible, tier 3 organs (ie non-favourably matched), are used locally. Mismatches for common HLA antigens should be avoided wherever possible, particularly in young recipients, to decrease the possible generation of HLA-specific antibodies reactive with a high proportion of potential donors. Such antibodies would make re-transplantation more difficult should the transplant fail.

8.32 A pre-transplant donor/recipient cross-match is a crucial procedure to prevent hyper-acute or accelerated transplant rejection. Each centre must therefore have an agreed and documented policy describing the cross-match tests to be performed prior to transplantation, the selection of samples to be tested and the interpretation of results. The policy must clearly define those circumstances in which pre-transplant cross-matching is not considered mandatory and this policy must be evidence based. Relevant sera from all patients on the current waiting lists must be stored and readily available for use in cross-match tests. The value of cross-matching by flow cytometry has been documented, particularly in recipients at high risk of rejection such as those with high levels of circulating antibody or a previous failed transplant.[29,30] Careful standardisation and quantification of the results are necessary.[31,32]

8.33   The laboratory must have a comprehensive screening programme for the detection and definition of HLA specific antibodies. Sensitised patients are those who have been exposed to HLA alloantigens through pregnancy, blood transfusion or a previous transplant and who have demonstrated an antibody response. The definition of sensitisation depends crucially upon the techniques used. The assay most widely used is the complement dependent cytotoxic assay using a panel of lymphocytes as target cells. Enzyme-linked immunosorbent assay (ELISA) and flow cytometric techniques are also commonly used.[33] The panel must be carefully selected to contain HLA specificities (HLA-A, -B, -Cw, -DR, -DQ) occurring in combinations that allow efficient interpretation of results. Non-HLA antibodies should be distinguished from those with specificity for HLA antigens. Although the degree of reactivity to the panel (panel reactivity antigen (PRA)) is often expressed as a percentage, this can be misleading since the panel is chosen to represent a wide range of antigens and not the population as a whole.

8.34   Complete definition of antibody specificity should be the goal of a screening programme since the failure to fully account for a patient's PRA in the specificities recognised by the antibody will adversely affect the points awarded by the national allocation programme. Assays used to detect allo-sensitisation must have a sensitivity equivalent to the cross-matching techniques used by the laboratory. Evidence of sensitisation in the form of circulating antibodies varies with time, so serum samples must be taken within two weeks of any blood transfusion, in the immediate post-transplant period, and in all patients on the transplant waiting list at least quarterly. Ideally, for female patients the HLA types of the father(s) of all pregnancies should be available. All HLA specificities against which the recipient reacts must be recorded as unacceptable antigens. Other known HLA antigens to which the recipient has previously been exposed may be considered unacceptable.

8.35   Conventionally, highly sensitised patients (HSPs) are defined as those who react with more than 85% of panel cells, despite the caveat in 8.32. To qualify as an HSP, the potential recipient must be shown to have antibodies specific for HLA alloantigens. Non-specific or auto-reactive IgM antibodies may give the impression of high panel reactivity, but since these antibodies do not prevent successful transplantation their presence must be carefully defined. However, IgM HLA-specific antibodies do occur, and may be deleterious, so simple *in vitro* destruction of IgM antibodies before testing is not recommended.[34] If antibody screening is carried out regularly after transplantation, accurate screening and cross-matching for re-transplantation can help achieve success rates after re-transplantation that are as high as those for first transplant.[33]

Immuno-suppressive regimens and early complications

RATIONALE

8.36 At the moment there are insufficient data to permit specific recommendations on the various immunosuppressive regimens involving monotherapy, double or triple therapy using prednisolone, azathioprine, cyclosporin microemulsion (Neoral™), tacrolimus, mycophenolate mofetil or rapamycin. Nor is the role of antibody therapies (basiliximab, dacluzimab, antilymphocyte globulin, OKT3 etc) clear. It is likely that mycophenolate mofetil, anti-CD25 antibodies and rapamycin will become increasingly used during the next few years because the number of early rejections using regimens which include these drugs appear to be lower, and lower rates of early rejection in turn are correlated with better long-term function and graft survival.

8.37 Graft survival rates appear to be similar with most of the regimens in current use, but graft survival is lower and rejection more common with regimens containing only prednisolone and azathioprine compared with those containing cyclosporin, and the other newer agents. Also, early rejection rates appear to be lower with the newer drugs (mycophenolate mofetil and tacrolimus). However, long-term experience may show that this beneficial effect is offset by more infections and other side effects. It is likely that a greater diversity of regimens will be used in future to 'tailor' therapy more specifically to individual patients' needs.

8.38 Newer agents such as mycophenolate and tacrolimus are still being assessed, and only further prospective studies will allow more precise recommendations to be made. Until these studies are completed, outcomes need careful auditing to allow accumulation of informative data. The choice of immunosuppressive regimen has substantial cost implications, which will need discussion with purchasers, but the high costs of a failed graft must also be borne in mind; cost effectiveness data are needed urgently in this area.

8.39 Renal transplant recipients are susceptible to opportunistic infections such as cytomegalovirus, pneumocystis and tuberculosis. The early detection of and/or prophylaxis against these infections in high-risk patients (eg cytomegalovirus (CMV) –ve recipient of a CMV +ve kidney) is possible, and their use must be judged taking into account potential hazards and expense. Guidelines on the prevention and treatment of cytomegalovirus infection transplant recipients have recently been published by the British Transplantation Society.[35]

8.40 Delayed graft function prolongs inpatient stay, increases the risk of renal vein thrombosis and may have an adverse effect on long-term outcome following recovery of renal function. Although evidence from prospective studies is lacking, strategies should be considered to minimise delayed function and to prevent renal venous thrombosis in susceptible patients.

Clinical outcome and audit

Standard

▶ Organs should be retrieved from at least 15 heart-beating donors per million population per year. Each unit should transplant at least 25 patients per million population per year using cadaver kidneys. Efforts should be made to limit the cold ischaemic time to less than 30 hours in all cases and to much less than 24 hours wherever possible. Each transplant unit which has appropriate resources to perform live donor transplantation should transplant a minimum of five living donor grafts per million population per year, but it is hoped that a higher number than this can be achieved in the future. At least 60% of recipients of cadaveric grafts should receive a 000 mismatch or other favourable matched kidney. (**Good practice**)

▶ At least 70% of heart-beating cadaver kidney transplants should function immediately, and at least 95% should function eventually. Graft survival of second grafts should be the same as for first grafts, provided that adequate analysis of alloantibodies and fluorescence activated cell sorter (FACS) cross-matching are used. There should be at least 95% patient survival at one year after transplantation for recipients of live donor and cadaveric kidneys. More than 85% of cadaver grafts and 90% of live grafts should still be working at one year and at least 66% of cadaver grafts and 73% of live donor grafts should still be working at five years. (**Good practice**)

RATIONALE

8.41   Clinical and medical audit should be an integral part of the work of the transplant unit. A list of items that should be regularly audited before and after transplantation is included in Appendix A. Patient survival, morbidity and transplant outcomes depend critically upon a number of case-mix factors such as the age and comorbidity of the population transplanted. This in turn depends upon the criteria for the selection process used among patients who are regarded as potential transplant recipients. It should be noted that transplant units have a legal responsibility to return the relevant Human Organ Transplant Act Forms (HOT A and HOT B) to UKT within seven days of the transplant procedure.

8.42   Data for outcomes of transplantation in the UK for 1996–8 are available in the renal transplant audit document published by the UKT (2000).[36] At the moment, recommended standards can be set for only some of the audit points for transplantation, for patients without major comorbidity and whose ages lie between 15 and 50 years of age. The figures suggested below are minimum acceptable results for cadaveric transplantation; clearly, if every unit in the UK were to achieve something near the present mean or better, the average standard would rise considerably. In 1996–8 the mean cadaver organ donor rate in the UK was 14 donors per million population per year while the mean figure for cadaver kidneys retrieved was 27 per million population. Lengthy cold ischaemic times (>30 hours) are associated with inferior graft survival in some studies,[37] and this is supported by data from the UK.[17]

8.43   For live donor transplants, the UK mean was four per million population in 1998, whilst in several European countries it was more than five per million population per annum, and in Norway exceeded 17 per million population per annum. The median waiting time on the cadaver transplant list in the UK is just under 500 days, but differs markedly for sensitised and non-sensitised patients, and is affected also by age, previous grafting and blood group. Policies vary from unit to unit as to which patients, and what proportion, are placed on transplant waiting lists, but the UK mean is 30% of the dialysis population. There will be variation according to the case-mix of patients on dialysis, and especially according to their comorbidity and age. In this area, equity and optimum use of the scarce resources of transplantable kidneys are in conflict. Currently, only 13% of recipients in the UK receive a 000 mismatch and 48% any other favourable match (see 8.29 for definition).

8.44 Table 3 shows the mean figures for the UK for first cadaver transplants performed from 1990 to 1997 and the recommended standards. It should be noted that these standards are based on outcome data, which do not take account of case-mix differences between different units.

Table 3. First cadaver transplants (UK, 1990–97) and recommended standards.

Survival time of patient	Mean UK survival (%)	Recommended minimum mean survival (%)
1 year	96	>95
5 years	88	>85

Survival time of graft*	Mean UK survival (%)	Recommended minimum mean survival (%)
1 year	85	>85
5 years	66	>66

*Graft failures include deaths with functioning grafts.

8.45 The mean rate of achieving immediate renal function following renal transplantation in the UK is around 70%, dependent upon the types of kidney accepted for use and their handling within the transplant unit. It is known that the kidneys that function immediately provide better long-term graft survival. In the UK 5% of kidneys never function.

8.46 It is much more difficult to set targets for transplant recipients with diabetes mellitus and/or other significant comorbidity, and we are working towards setting standards for such patients in the future. It should be noted that at the time of writing a draft DH document is being prepared which may have more ambitious targets for cadaveric and live donor numbers.

Paediatric section

Definitions

8.47 The term 'paediatric recipient' refers to children and adolescents under the age of 18 years, regardless of whether they are being managed in paediatric or adult transplant units. This includes infants and children (up to fifteenth birthday as defined by the British Association for Paediatric Nephrology (BAPN)) and adolescents (15–18 years).[38]

Access to transplantation and allocation of kidneys

Standards

▶ All children under 15 years of age being prepared for or undergoing transplantation should be cared for in a paediatric nephrology, dialysis and transplant centre. (**Good practice**)

▶ The UKT scheme giving priority to children for favourably matched kidneys should continue. **(Good practice)**

▶ Pre-emptive transplantation should be encouraged as it conserves peritoneal and vascular access for future use and improves growth. **(Good practice)**

▶ Living related donor transplantation should be encouraged. **(Good practice)**

8.48 All discussions about transplantation should take place between the relevant professionals (transplant surgeon, paediatric nephrologist and representatives of the multi-professional team) and the parents/guardians, in the presence of the child where age-appropriate. The benefits and risks associated with living donor transplantation and the risks of transplantation, including infection and malignant disease, should be discussed and supported by written information. Checklists should be used to ensure and document that all of the relevant issues, including infection and malignant disease, have been covered. This exercise should be repeated 6–12 monthly for those who have not undergone transplantation.

8.49 The current UKT allocation algorithm gives priority to paediatric recipients for all 000 mismatched and all favourably matched organs, irrespective of whether the donor is paediatric or adult. (Adult centres may register small adults (<35 kg) as paediatric at their discretion.) In light of the small recipient pool, the problems associated with maintaining dialysis access and optimising growth in small children with end stage renal failure, it is essential that this system of prioritisation continues. All children with end stage renal failure should be on the waiting list for transplantation unless there are relative contraindications, such as the increased graft loss associated with transplantation in small children (Table 4).

8.50 The transplantation of kidneys into children with renal failure prior to the commencement of dialysis (pre-emptive transplantation) results in improved growth and psychosocial development, and conserves peritoneal and haemodialysis access for future use in childhood or adult life. It is therefore widely used within paediatric transplant units. Furthermore, the long-term outcome for pre-emptive transplants may be superior to that of transplants performed in children established on dialysis.[39,40] A child is generally considered for pre-emptive transplantation once the GFR had fallen to below 15 ml/min/1.73 m^2, and either dialysis is anticipated within 18–24 months and/or an important complication of renal failure is present, eg growth failure. With very young or small children, the clinician and family have to consider the balance between the benefits of pre-emptive transplantation, the particular difficulties associated with the provision of dialysis (access problems, poor developmental outcome etc), and the increased graft loss associated with transplantation in this high-risk population. The associated increased requirement for donor organs which pre-emptive transplantation produces should be met by the active promotion of living related donor (LRD) transplantation.

Table 4. One-year UK and Ireland paediatric graft survival data 1986–95. Source: UKT.

Recipient age (years)	Number	% Survival	95% CI
0–2	29	62	44–80
2–5	160	69	62–76
5–10	284	70	65–75
10–15	426	81	77–84
15–18	309	75	70–80

Donor age (years)	Number	% Survival	95% CI
0–2	30	47	29–65
2–5	178	58	51–66
5–10	284	75	70–80
10–15	248	79	74–84
15–18	94	88	82–95
18–35	221	81	75–86
36+	153	76	70–83

HLA mismatch	Number	% Survival	95% CI
000	55	84	74–93
Favourable	232	82	77–87
Other 0 DR	132	75	68–82
1 DR	634	75	72–79
2 DR	155	58	50–66

Cold ischaemia time (hours)	Number	% Survival	95% CI
0–15	113	87	80–93
15–20	161	89	85–94
20–25	194	79	74–84
25–30	96	78	69–85
30 +	95	76	67–84

CI = confidence interval

Organ donation/ living donor transplantation

Recommendation

▶ The use of kidneys from donors under the age of five years or over 55 years is not recommended in paediatric patients. **(B)**

8.51   The use of kidneys from children under five years of age is associated with a poor long-term outcome for the graft, particularly where such kidneys are used in small recipients (Table 4).[41,42] The use of such kidneys should therefore be avoided in paediatric recipients: a number of adult units may utilise the organs for 'en-bloc' transplantation into adult recipients. The use of kidneys from older adult donors is also associated with poor long-term graft survival (Table 4), and therefore only kidneys from cadaver donors under 50–55 years of age should be offered to paediatric recipients. The living donor transplantation rate in UK paediatric centres is significantly lower than that in other European countries and North America. Major steps need to be taken to redress this situation in view of the significantly improved outcome of living donor compared with cadaveric transplantation[43] and the flexibility which the procedure offers the family. Units must provide families with information about these benefits. Efforts should be made to limit cold ischaemia time (Table 4).

The transplant unit

Recommendation

▶ There should be 24-hour access to a consultant paediatric nephrologist, transplant surgeon, urologist, general surgeon, anaesthetist and intensivist. (**Good practice**)

8.52   There are 13 paediatric nephrology centres in the UK, 11 of which undertake renal transplantation.[38] All children under 15 years of age should be transplanted in these units in view of their special needs, the provision of appropriate support services and maintenance of expertise. Because of the delay in physical and emotional maturation that often characterises chronic renal failure, and the particular problems associated with non-adherence in adolescents, many 15–18 year olds are most appropriately transplanted within paediatric centres.

8.53   Paediatric transplant units should in general serve at least a two million total population. Units should be affiliated to and work closely with adult transplant units performing at least 50 transplants per annum. At least 20% of transplants performed should be from living donors. Future national planning of transplantation might give consideration to some concentration of expertise in the larger centres, and there should certainly be no increase in the number of centres undertaking paediatric renal transplantation.

8.54   Children undergoing renal transplantation should have 24-hour access to a consultant paediatric nephrologist, transplant surgeon, paediatric surgeon/urologist, paediatric anaesthetist and paediatric intensivist. All treatment modalities for renal failure should exist on site, along with specialist paediatric nurses, dieticians, child mental health specialists (child psychiatrist and/or child psychologist), social workers, teachers and play therapists. Such psychosocial care for the child and their family should have continuity between the pre- and post-transplant period.[38,44] Centres should be expected to implement the Department of Health guidelines, *The welfare of young children in hospital* (1991).[45]

8.55   Cadaveric transplantation should be performed in the paediatric transplant unit even if it is geographically distinct from their affiliated transplant centre: this will require flexibility on the part of both transplant surgeons and paediatric surgeons, and theatre staff in the paediatric centres. Living donors should always be managed within adult institutions to ensure donor safety: this will necessitate the transportation of donor organs to paediatric centres where these are geographically distinct. Where living related donor transplantation occurs, the non-donor parent should have unrestricted access to both donor and recipient. With good models of care, early transfer to non-transplanting paediatric nephrology centres nearer the patient's home is appropriate for long term follow-up. All paediatric renal transplant recipients should be registered with the national Paediatric Renal Registry regardless of whether they are managed in adult or paediatric centres.

Histocompatibility matching and allocation of donor kidneys

Recommendation

▶ Centres should aim for at least 60% of kidneys being favourably matched. **(B)**

8.56 In view of the increased long-term survival of zero mismatched and favourably matched grafts, and the significant problems associated with the sensitisation of children following the loss of less well-matched grafts, centres should aim for at least 60% of kidneys being favourably matched. However, UKT have a calculated 'matchability score' for each paediatric recipient that can be used to assess the likely length of time before a 000 or favourably matched kidney becomes available. This could be used to guide acceptance of a particular kidney for a particular child. For those very likely to receive a well-matched kidney reasonably soon, there is every incentive to avoid transplantation of a mismatched kidney in order to avoid subsequent sensitisation. Conversely, for those patients highly unlikely to receive a well-matched kidney, acceptance of the first suitable kidney may avoid an undue wait on the transplant waiting-list.

Immuno-suppressive regimens and early complications

Recommendation

▶ Centres should be encouraged to enter patients into prospective randomised paediatric trials to assess the efficacy, safety and tolerability of new immunosuppressive agents. **(Good practice)**

8.57 There are insufficient data to permit specific recommendations to be made with regard to immunosuppressive therapy. Cyclosporine-based triple therapy remains the most widely used combination of agents. Data from the North American Pediatric Renal Transplant Cooperative Study show an increasing tendency in North American centres to use newer immunosuppressive agents.[46] It is essential that the efficacy, safety and tolerability of these agents are fully assessed in prospective randomised paediatric trials and all centres should be encouraged to enter patients into such trials. Given the improved results obtained with the use of well-matched cadaveric transplants, the widespread adoption of intensive immunosuppressive regimens may not be justified.[41] More potent immunosuppressive therapies may be associated with an increased lifetime risk of malignancy, which is particularly important with paediatric patients who have many years of renal replacement therapy ahead of them. Immunosuppressive regimens need to be tailored to paediatric patients. It is not acceptable to extrapolate the findings of adult-based studies to the childhood population.

8.58 Non-compliance remains a major cause of graft loss in the paediatric (specifically adolescent) population[47–50] and drugs which are complex to administer or are associated with adverse cosmetic side-effects will increase the non-compliance rate.[50] Growth post-transplantation may be enhanced by the use of corticosteroids on an alternate day basis, and units should strive to achieve this within six months post-transplantation if clinical circumstances permit.

Transfer of patients to adult service

Recommendation

▶ All centres should have a written policy for the transfer of adolescents to adult units. (**Good practice**)

8.59   The transfer to an adult unit is a time of great stress to many patients and their families. A formal transfer policy requiring close liaison with local adult transplant units should exist. The patient's paediatric record should be summarised for the adult team taking over care. Age at transfer should vary according to circumstance: many units will transfer patients on completion of secondary education or at age 18, whichever is the earlier. The long-term follow-up of young adults over 18 years of age within paediatric units is undesirable.

Clinical outcome and audit

Standards

▶ Each unit should report their data to the Paediatric Renal Registry to enable annual national assessment of outcomes of paediatric transplantation. (**Good epidemiological practice**)

▶ Centres should audit each graft loss to identify possible avoidable factors. (**Good practice**)

8.60   Because of a combination of immunological, technical and other factors, paediatric graft survival is inferior to that of adults, and the application of standards based upon adult survival data to children is inappropriate. UKT has recently analysed the outcome of kidneys transplanted into paediatric recipients between 1986 and 1995 (Table 4). At present only unifactoral one-year graft and patient survival data are available. Centres should currently aim to have better graft survival than that reported between 1986 and 1995. The small number of paediatric transplants performed in many centres further complicates statistical analysis. In addition to individual unit outcome assessment, there should be an annual national assessment of outcomes of paediatric transplantation, with each graft loss being examined to identify possible avoidable factors. Audit data (Appendix A) should be collected for paediatric recipients whether they are managed in adult or paediatric units.

References

1   McMillan MA, Briggs JD. Survey of selection for cadaveric renal transplantation in the United Kingdom. *Nephrol Dial Transplant* 1995;**10**:855–8.

2   Mange KC, Joffe MM, Feldman HI. Effect of the use or non use of long term dialysis on the subsequent survival of renal transplants from living donors. *N Engl J Med* 2001;**344**:726–31.

3   Kasike BL, Ramos EL, Gaston RS *et al*. The evaluation of renal transplant candidates: clinical practice guidelines. Patient care and education committee of the American Society of Transplant Physicians. *J Am Soc Nephrol* 1995;**6**:1–34.

4   The EBPG expert group on renal transplantation. European Best Practice Guidelines for Renal Transplantation. *Nephrol Dial Transplant* 2000;**15**:suppl 7.

5   Cameron JS, Crompton F, Koffman G, Bewick M. Transplantation in elderly recipients. *Geriatr Nephrol Urol* 1994;**4**:93–9.

6   Cantarovich D, Baatard R, Baranger T *et al.* Cadaveric renal transplantation after 60 years of age: a single centre experience. *Transpl Int* 1994;**7**:33–8.

7   Woo YM, Jardine AG, Clark AF *et al.* Early graft function and patient survival following cadaveric renal transplantation. *Kidney Int* 1999;**55**:692–9.

8   Schnuelle P, Lorenz D, Trede M, Van der Woude FJ. Impact of renal cadaveric transplantation on survival in end stage renal failure: evidence for reduced mortality risk compared with haemodialysis during long term follow up. *J Am Soc Nephrol* 1998;**9**:2135–41.

9   Wolfe RA, Ashby VB, Milford EL *et al.* Comparison of mortality in all patients on dialysis, patients on dialysis awaiting transplantation, and recipients of a first cadaveric transplant. *N Engl J Med* 1999; **341**:1725–30.

10 Wight C, Cohen B. Shortage of organs for transplantation: crisis measures must include better detection and maintenance of donors. *Br Med J* 1996;**312**:989–90.

11 New W, Solomon M, Dingwall R, McHale J. *A question of give and take: improving the supply of donor organs for transplantation.* London: King's Fund Institute, 1994.

12 Falvey S, Morgan V. Transplant coordinators need more money for education. *Br Med J* 1996;**312**: 1358 (letter).

13 Terasaki PI, Cecka JM, Gjertson DW, Takemoto S. High survival rates of kidney transplants from spousal and living unrelated donors. *N Engl J Med* 1995;**333**:333–6.

14 Fehrman-Ekholm I, Elinder CG, Stenbeck M *et al.* Kidney donors live longer. *Transplantation* 1997; **64**:976–8.

15 British Transplantation Society/Renal Association working party. *United Kingdom guidelines for living donor kidney transplantation.* London: British Transplantation Society/Renal Association, 2000.

16 Sutherland DER, Stratta RJ, Gruessner AC. Pancreas outcome by recipient category: single pancreas versus combined kidney-pancreas. *Cur Opin Organ Transplant* 1998;**3**:231–41.

17 Morris PJ, Johnson RJ, Fuggle SV *et al.* Analysis of factors that affect outcome of primary cadaveric renal transplantation in the UK. *Lancet* 1999:**354**:1147–52.

18 Scottish Intercollegiate Guidelines Network. *Lipids and the primary prevention of coronary artery disease.* Edinburgh: Royal College of Physicians of Edinburgh, 1999.

19 Scottish Intercollegiate Guidelines Network. *Secondary prevention of coronary heart disease following myocardial infarction.* Edinburgh: SIGN, 2000.

20 Kew CE, Curtis JJ 2000; 11. Cardiovascular disease in renal transplant recipients. *Cur Opin Organ Transplant* 1998;**3**:183–7.

21 Silkensen JR. Long term complications in renal transplantation. *J Am Soc Nephrol* 2000;**11**:582–8.

22 Royal College of Physicians of London. *Osteoporosis: clinical guidelines for prevention and treatment; update.* London: RCP, 2000.

23 Rodger RSC, Watson MJ, Sellars L *et al.* Hypothalmic – pituitary – adrenocortical suppression and recovery in renal transplant patients returning to maintenance dialysis. *Q J Med* 1986;**61**:1039–46.

24 Gregor PJ, Kramer P, Weimer W, Van Saase JL. Infections after renal allograft failure in patients with or without low dose maintenance immunosuppression. *Transplantation* 1997;**63**:1528–30.

25 Department of Health. *Review of renal services in England 1993–4.* London: NHS Executive, 1996.

26 Royal Surgical Colleges Senate. Consultant surgical practice and training in the United Kingdom. London, Royal Surgical Colleges Senate, 1997.

27 Held PJ, Kahan BD, Hunsicher LG *et al.* The impact of HLA mismatches on the survival of first cadaver kidney transplants. *N Engl J Med* 1994;**331**:765–70.

28   Opelz G (for the Collaborative Transplant Study). Influence of treatment with cyclosporin, azathioprine and steroids on chronic allograft failure. *Kidney Int* 1995;**48**(Suppl 52):s89–92.

29   Bryan CF, Baier KA, Nelson PW *et al.* Long-term graft survival is improved in cadaveric renal retransplantation by flow cytometric cross-matching. *Transplantation* 1998;**66**:1827–32.

30   Martin S, Liggett H, Robson A *et al.* The association between a positive T and B cell flow cytometry cross-match and renal transplant failure. *Transpl Immunol* 1993;**1**:270–6.

31   Harmer AW, Garner S, Bell AE *et al.* Evaluation of the flow cytometric cross-match. Preliminary results of a multicentre study. *Transplantation* 1996;**61**:1108–11.

32   Shenton BK, Bell AE, Harmer AW *et al.* Importance of methodology in the flow cytometric cross-match: a multicentre study. *Transplant Proc* 1997;**29**:1454–5.

33   Martin S, Taylor CJ. The immunologically sensitised renal transplant recipient: the impact of advances in technology on organ allocation and transplant outcome. *Transplant Rev* 1999;**13**:40–51.

34   Taylor CJ, Chapman JR, Ting A, Morris AJ. Characterisation of lymphocytotoxic antibodies causing a positive cross-match in renal transplantation. *Transplantation* 1989;**48**:953–8.

35   British Transplantation Society. *Guidelines for the prevention and management of cytomegalovirus disease after solid organ transplantation.* London: BTS, 2002.

36   United Kingdom Transplant Service Special Authority. *Renal Transplant Audit, 1996-8.* Bristol: UKT, 2000.

37   Cecka JM, Cho YW, Terasaki PI. Analyses of the UNOS scientific renal transplant registry at three years: early events affecting transplant success. *Transplantation* 1992;**53**:59–64.

38   British Association for Paediatric Nephrology. *The provision of services in the United Kingdom for children and adolescents with renal disease.* Report of a Working Party of the British Association for Paediatric Nephrology. London: BAPN, 1995.

39   Vats AN, Donaldson L, Fine RN, Chavers BM. Pretransplant dialysis and outcome of renal transplantation in North American children: a NAPRTCS Study. *Transplantation* 2000;**7**:1414–19.

40   Mahmoud A, Said M-H, Dawahra M, Hadj-Aissa A, Schnell M *et al.* Outcome of pre-emptive renal transplantation and pretransplantation dialysis in children. *Pediatr Nephrol* 1997;**11**:537–41.

41   Postlethwaite RJ. Paediatric renal transplantation in the United Kingdom and Ireland 1986–1995. *Pediatr Transplant*, in press.

42   Tejani AH, Stablein DM, Sullivan EK, Alexander SR, Fine RN, Harmon WE, Kohaut EC. The impact of donor source, recipient age, pre-operative immunotherapy and induction therapy on early and late acute rejections in children: a report of the North American Pediatric Renal Transplant Cooperative Study (NAPRTCS). *Pediatr Transplant* 1998;**2**:318–24.

43   Benfield MR, McDonald R, Sullivan EK, Stablein DM, Tejani A. The 1997 annual renal transplantation in children report of the North American Pediatric Renal Transplant Cooperative Study. *Pediatr Transplant* 1999;**3**:152–67.

44   Davis ID, Bunchman TE, Grimm PC, Benfield MR, Briscoe DM, Harmon WE, Alexander SR, Avner ED. Pediatric renal transplantation: indications and special considerations. A position paper from the American Society of Transplant Physicians. *Pediatr Transplant* 1998;**2**:117–29.

45   Department of Health. *The welfare of young children in hospital.* London: DH, 1991.

46   Benfield MR, Stablein D, Tejani A. Trends in immunosuppressive therapy: a report of the North American Pediatric Renal Transplant Cooperative Study. *Pediatr Transplant* 1999;**3**:27–32.

47   Gagnadoux MF, Niaudet P, Broyer M Non-immunological risk factors in paediatric renal transplantation *Pediatr Nephrol* 1993;**7**:89–95.

48   Korsch BM, Fine RN, Negrete VF. Non-compliance in children with renal transplants. *Pediatr Nephrol* 1978;**61**:872–6.

49   Ettenger RB, Rosenthal JT, Marik JL, Malekadeh MH, Forsythe SB, Kamil ES, Fine RN. Improved cadaveric renal transplant outcome in children. *Pediatr Nephrol* 1991;**5**:137–42.

50   Meyers KE, Weiland H, Thomson PD. Paediatric renal transplant non-compliance. *Pediatr Nephrol* 1995;**9**:189–92.

9 Blood-borne viruses and microbiology in the renal unit

Microbiological services

9.1   This chapter, which applies to both adults and children, deals mainly with aspects of cross-infection in and between patients and staff. It should be noted that results, especially those of tests for blood-borne viruses (BBVs), will be needed out of hours, and rapidly; this requires collaboration and discussion with local microbiologists.

Blood-borne viruses

9.2   In 1972 the Rosenheim Advisory Group issued good practice guidelines to prevent the transmission of hepatitis B virus (HBV) in dialysis and transplantation units.[1] New BBVs, including particularly hepatitis C virus (HCV) and human immunodeficiency virus (HIV) have been identified since then, but separate guidance has not been issued. Further BBVs such as hepatitis G have been identified.[2–4] Although their carriage rate is greater in patients on dialysis than in the general population, their clinical significance – especially in the long term – remains unclear.

9.3   Universal precautions accepted against viral transmission, designed both for the protection of the staff and to prevent cross-infection between patients, are an essential discipline in dealing with dialysis patients. All patients with either chronic renal failure (CRF) or acute renal failure (ARF) should be managed as if they were chronic virus carriers until they have been fully tested. Regular testing is part of the subsequent management of patients and the running of renal units. Staff training should incorporate and emphasise precautions against BBVs. Where available and effective, immunisation should be offered to staff; there is evidence that in the case of HBV this has not been widely practised in the UK.[5]

9.4   In May 1995, the Department of Health (DH) asked the Public Health Laboratory Service (PHLS) to prepare advice, in the form of draft guidelines, on the precautions that should be taken in renal units to prevent the transmission of BBVs in general. A working party was set up which included representatives of the Royal College of Physicians and the Royal College of Pathologists. Their document was submitted to the DH in late 1996 and is currently under review. When the DH makes its comprehensive report, its recommendations will become the norm.

Good working practices

> ### *Recommendation*
>
> ▶ The general and universal precautions described below should be observed. (**Good practice**)

RATIONALE

9.5   Transmission of HBV, HCV and HIV to staff or patients may occur as a result of percutaneous exposure to blood or other body fluids. Viruses may also be transmitted directly to mucosal surfaces or patient tissues through droplets, via the hands or forearms of staff, or indirectly through contaminated equipment or supplies. Great care should be exercised when treating all patients and all procedures should be reviewed regularly as part of local risk assessment in collaboration with the hospital infection control team.

9.6   These guidelines should be read in conjunction with all other good practice guidelines which are relevant to maintaining safety in renal units; these include *Protection against blood-borne infections in the workplace: HIV and hepatitis* (Advisory Committee on Dangerous Pathogens (ACDP))[6] and *Guidance for clinical healthcare workers: protection against blood-borne virus infections* (Expert Advisory Group on AIDS, and the Advisory Group on Hepatitis).[7] Guidance for ensuring the safety of transplanted organs is given in *Guidance on the microbiological safety of human tissues, organs and cells used in transplantation* (Advisory Committee on the Microbiological Safety of Blood and Tissues for Transplantation).[8]

9.7   The working environment of a renal unit should be conducive to good clinical practice with adequate lighting and layout, incorporating sufficient space between patient stations. There should be a plentiful supply of protective clothing including gloves, aprons, visors, and sharps containers. Gloves and aprons should be changed after attending to each patient. It is recommended that there should be one hand basin for every three dialysis stations and one hand basin for each isolated or segregated area, and that hand-washing should be performed with antiseptic scrub before attending to each patient. Alcohol-based hand wipes are not recommended for routine hand hygiene between patient contacts in a haemodialysis (HD) unit. Surfaces of dialysis machines and other parts of the station, eg shelving, bed table etc, should be washed with soap and water between patient sessions and disinfected daily with chlorine-based disinfectant (1,000 ppm chlorine) or some suitable alternative, when stations are used by more than one patient. Daily cleaning of dialysis units is imperative to eliminate dirt, grime and grease.

9.8   There must be adequate skin protection for staff working in HD units, and staff with chronic skin problems should seek occupational health advice regarding their suitability to work in a renal unit. Staff should only eat or drink in designated staff rest areas. When working in the unit, domestic staff should wear aprons and gloves, which should be discarded before leaving the area. Units should work towards eliminating the use of multi-use vials. Blood spillages should be dealt with by fully trained staff. Small spillages should be wiped up with a paper towel saturated in a chlorine-based disinfectant (10,000 ppm chlorine). Large spillages should either be covered with dichloroisocyanate granules and left for two minutes before cleaning up with paper towels, or gently flooded with hypochlorite solution, left for two minutes before thoroughly cleaning with water and detergent. Clinical waste should be bagged before being taken out of the segregated BBV area. Used HD and continuous ambulatory peritoneal dialysis (CAPD) fluids should be disposed directly to a drain or sluice.

9.9   Action to be taken in the event of transmission of BBVs is outlined in 9.12. Other measures include stopping elective transfer of patients to other units and notification of any unit of an outbreak of BBV infection if a transfer has taken place in the previous three months. Consideration should be given to placing patients infected with BBV on home HD, CAPD or, in a case of HCV, considered for a renal transplant.

Immunisation and patient testing

Recommendations

▶ Patients awaiting the start of end stage renal disease (ESRD) treatment should be immunised against HBV as soon as possible while their plasma creatinine remains relatively low. **(B)**

▶ All long-term dialysis patients should be immunised against HBV. Those who develop an adequate antibody response should be given a booster dose of vaccine every five years. As there is evidence that poor responders derive some benefit from vaccination, they should be given a booster after one year and every five years thereafter. Non-responders should receive a repeat course of vaccine. **(B)**

▶ Testing should be carried out three monthly for hepatitis B surface antigen (HBsAg), and HCV antibody and annually for HIV antibody. An annual test for HBsAg is sufficient for patients who have demonstrated immunity. More frequent testing is appropriate in those exposed to BBV (see below). **(Good practice)**

▶ Hepatitis B immunoglobulin and vaccine should be given, if appropriate, to susceptible patients who have been exposed to the virus. **(B)**

▶ The patient's informed consent to testing should be obtained. Those who withhold consent or who are incapable of giving consent should be managed as though they were BBV infected. However, infected patients should not be denied dialysis. **(Good practice)**

RATIONALE

Immunisation against HBV

9.10   Although the prevalence of HBV is low among dialysis patients in the UK, and the risk of transmission is correspondingly low, the environment of a renal unit predisposes to blood borne viral cross-infection, and every attempt should be made to immunise patients against HBV. Although antibody response is reduced after standard (20 µg) doses of Hep B vaccine (Engerix B), immunisation rates may be improved with double dosing of the vaccine or the use of other vaccines such as HB vax PRO (Aventis) when antibody levels of >100 mlU/ml in 70 to 80% of immunised patients have been described. Hepatitis B vaccination is particularly important for patients visiting units overseas, especially Africa, India and the Far East. There is a higher response rate in patients pending dialysis[9] and immunisation against hepatitis B should be standard practice in low renal clearance clinics. A joint approach with the patient's general practitioner (GP) using a shared-care protocol may be set up with the GP responsible for administering the vaccine.

Response to immunisation

9.11   Following a course of immunisation at 0, 1, and 6 months, antibody levels should be checked 2–4 months after the last dose of vaccine. Patients developing an anti HBs level of 100 mlU/ml or more should be given a booster dose at five years; poor responders (anti HBs levels of between 10 and 100 mlU/ml) should be given a booster dose after one and five years. Non-responders (antibody levels of <10 mlU/ml) should receive a repeat course of vaccine.*

*There is continuing debate amongst virologists about the level of antibody response which protects against infection with hepatitis B. In future a positive antibody level may be all that is required and booster doses may become unnecessary. Please consult with local virological departments for up-to-date information.

9.12   Although the frequency of testing for BBV amongst patients on HD has varied in renal units in the past, it is suggested that regular surveillance is essential to alert renal unit staff to any possible outbreaks. HBsAg, HCV Ab and HIV should be tested before the patient starts or restarts HD. Immunosuppressed transplant patients who are HCV antibody negative and are returning to dialysis should be screened for HCV ribonucleic acid (RNA) before dialysis. HIV positive patients should also be screened for HCV RNA. HBsAg and HCV Ab should be tested three monthly and HIV annually, and prior to establishment on a renal transplant list. Patients with anti-HBs levels of more than 100 mIU/ml need only be tested for HBsAg annually. More frequent tests will be necessary in the following situations:

▶   When a previously unrecognised case of BBV infection occurs, other patients who have shared the same dialysis session *or have used the same machine* should be screened for the virus concerned. If the risk is HBV, patients who have not demonstrated adequate immunity to HBV in the preceding 12 months (anti-HBs <100 mIU/ml) should be screened weekly for three months, given a booster dose of vaccine and given HB Ig if the anti-HBs is <10 mlU/ml. The newly-infected patient should be dialysed in a separate area using a dedicated machine, if infected with HBV. If a new case of HCV is found, it is suggested that a test for hepatitis C RNA is obtained for those patients who have shared the same dialysis session, and specialist advice requested about the need for further tests.

▶   Any patient who develops abnormal liver function tests should be screened for hepatitis B and C.

▶   Patients who use dialysis facilities outside the UK should be encouraged to be immunised against hepatitis B. On their return they should be tested for HBV and HCV preferably before receiving dialysis in their own renal unit and should be treated as potentially infected. A test for HBsAg should be carried out every two weeks for three months on patients who have anti-HBs levels of <100 mlU/ml. A dedicated machine should be used until the risk of HBV infection is discounted. Patients who have dialysed in another UK renal unit adhering to these standards do not need isolation or use of a dedicated machine providing they have not been accidentally exposed to BBV whilst in the other unit.

Management of patients carrying BBVs

Recommendations

▶ Whenever possible, staff should care for only BBV-infected or uninfected patients during one shift. If this is not practicable, the more experienced staff should be assigned the task of caring for a mixed group of patients. Designated staff should nurse affected patients when there has been an outbreak of BBV infection in a unit. In the case of hepatitis B, staff who demonstrated immunity should care for the patients whenever possible. (**Good practice**)

▶ Carriers of hepatitis B should be dialysed in separate rooms on dedicated machines. (**Good practice**)

▶ Carriers of hepatitis C should be dialysed in separate shifts and units should move towards providing separate rooms for such patients. (**Good practice**)

▶ Dialysis machines used for patients positive for hepatitis C may be used for other patients provided that the dialysis circuit has been adequately decontaminated and the external surface cleaned with some suitable disinfectant between patient use. (**Good practice**)

▶ Segregation of HIV infected patients should be considered, based on local risk assessment. Their machines should be treated as for patients with hepatitis C. (**Good practice**)

RATIONALE

HBV

9.13   Although universal precautions are appropriate against all BBVs, hepatitis B is much more infective than either HIV or hepatitis C. Patients carrying hepatitis B should have dedicated dialysis monitors and be isolated in a separate room within the dialysis unit; nursing traffic between these two areas should be reduced to a minimum. There is no evidence indicating whether or not patients should be segregated while being transported to and from the dialysis unit.

HCV and HIV

9.14   There are different views on the isolation of patients and machines in patients who are carriers of hepatitis C. Nosocomial transmission of hepatitis C can undoubtedly occur, but the mode of transmission is often unclear.[10] Both 'horizontal' transmission of virus between patients not sharing a machine[11] and 'vertical' transmission among patients sharing a machine have been described.[12] The Public Health Laboratory Service (PHLS) working party felt that horizontal transmission is more likely to occur than vertical transmission and that patients who are hepatitis C antibody positive should be treated in segregated areas of the dialysis unit, but not on dedicated machines. This advice may be relatively easy to implement in dialysis units with few patients with BBVs, but rather more difficult when a number of patients with HBV or HCV are involved, and even more difficult if isolation facilities are required for patients who are methicillin resistant staphylococcus aureus (MRSA) or vancomycin resistant enterococcus (VRE) positive. For this reason renal units may wish to prioritise patient isolation in the limited space available. Although difficult at present, units should work towards the availability of separate rooms for patients with HCV, MRSA and VRE carriage. Great importance is attached to the maintenance of strict universal precautions when dealing with all patients, not just those who are positive for BBV, including frequent hand washing, and use of gloves and aprons, which should be discarded between attending to different patients.

Dialysis equipment

9.15   The design of modern dialysis machines makes them an unlikely source of cross-infection of BBV. The manufacturers' recommendations for assembly and use of equipment should always be followed. The entire dialysis fluid circuit should be decontaminated after each use, by heat or chemical disinfection. The external surface should be wiped over between each patient use using a chlorine-based disinfectant (1,000 ppm) or some suitable alternative. Units should not reuse dialysers from patients carrying a BBV which would expose staff to the risk of infection and would require separate reuse facilities.

Dialysis personnel and BBVs

Standards

▶ Staff working in dialysis units in contact with patients, machines or materials used in dialysis should show immunity to HBV. Non-, or poor, responders should be tested annually for HBs antigen and antibody to HB core antigen. Staff who are positive for HBsAg should demonstrate they are not HBe antigen positive or are HBe antigen negative with a viral load of less than 10^3 genome equivalents per ml. Non-clinical staff need not be tested for BBVs. (**Good practice**)

continued

▶ There is no need to screen for HCV or HIV in staff, but those known to be at risk of acquiring infection or known to be infected should be encouraged to seek advice from an occupational health physician. (**Good practice**)

HBV

9.16   It is now a pre-requisite that all staff working in a dialysis unit should show immunity against HBV, or be offered immunisation before employment. Poor or non-responders to hepatitis B immunisation should not be debarred from working in a dialysis unit. Although the activities undertaken by staff are not considered exposure-prone procedures (as defined by the DH), transmission of BBVs from staff to patients cannot be entirely ruled out and staff who are positive for HBsAg should demonstrate they are not HBe antigen positive or are HBe antigen negative with a viral load of less than 10^3 genome equivalents per ml. Non-clinical staff need not be tested for BBVs.

HCV and HIV

9.17   There are no regulations governing the employment of staff positive for HCV or HIV in renal units. Nevertheless, staff who know they are positive for hepatitis C or HIV, should seek advice about limitations to their practice from an occupational health physician. Confidentiality should be maintained at all times. Family and other carers actively involved in dialysis should be considered in the same way as unit staff.

Role of occupational health departments and infectious disease control team

9.18   It is imperative that dialysis units have a designated safety officer and safety committee and easy access to occupational health departments and the infectious disease control team when dealing with outbreaks of BBVs and staffing matters relevant to the acquisition of BBVs.

Patients on CAPD and those not yet on dialysis

Patients treated by CAPD

9.19   Patients starting continuous ambulatory peritoneal dialysis (CAPD) should be screened for BBVs at the start of treatment. They should also be encouraged to be immunised against hepatitis B, as it is likely that they will need HD in the short or longer term. There are no recommendations about the periodic testing for BBVs, but screening annually or before putting a patient on a transplant list would seem appropriate. Patients on peritoneal dialysis (PD) with BBVs that are admitted to hospital do not need isolation, but all body fluids including PD fluid should be handled with care. Universal precautions should be sufficient to avoid cross-infection from and to patients on CAPD while in hospital (eg for training or owing to peritonitis); we do not recommend that these patients be isolated in separate rooms.

BBVs and patients in CRF not yet on dialysis

9.20   Precautions should be observed for patients in CRF not yet on dialysis in exactly the same way as for those on dialysis. Testing for BBVs should be routine in those entering CRF (low clearance) clinics, but it is not possible yet to recommend whether or how often this should be repeated. As noted above, immunisation for HBV is best carried out in the CRF clinic.

9.21   Following advice from the Advisory Committee on Dangerous Pathogens and the Spongiform Encephalopathy Advisory Committee Joint Working Group on Transmissible Spongiform Encephalopathies, it appears that the risk of transmission of Creutzfeld-Jakob disease (CJD) from HD machines is minimal providing the equipment is correctly maintained. The issue of dialyser reuse and CJD is currently under discussion with the DH. Patients suspected of being infected with CJD should be dialysed on a separate machine.[13]

Staphylococcus aureus (SA) infection control in dialysis units

Recommendations

▶ All units should have a documented infection control policy covering general measures together with specific advice on limiting SA-related infections and preventing the spread of MRSA and other multi-resistant strains. This will usually be developed in conjunction with the hospital infection control unit. Key features should include guidelines for screening to detect nasal carriage, prophylactic therapy in different dialysis populations, antibiotic therapy for presumed *staphylococcal* infections, staff and patient education, an emphasis on the importance of hand washing and an isolation policy for MRSA carriers admitted to hospital.

▶ All dialysis patients should be screened on a three-monthly basis for SA nasal carriage. **(Good practice)**

▶ Patients undergoing HD via a temporary central venous dialysis catheter should have either 2% mupirocin ointment **(A)** or povidone-iodine ointment **(A)** applied to the cannula exit site after insertion and at the end of each dialysis session.

▶ All HD patients who are SA nasal carriers should receive either eradication therapy with a course of intranasal 2% mupirocin cream **(Good practice)** or eradication therapy followed by long-term once-weekly application of 2% mupirocin cream. **(A)**

▶ Patients on PD should apply 2% mupirocin ointment to the exit site on a daily or alternate daily basis as part of routine exit-site care. **(B)**

▶ Patients on PD who are SA nasal carriers should receive either eradication therapy with a course of intranasal 2% mupirocin cream **(Good practice)** or have regular five-day courses of intranasal 2% mupirocin every four weeks. **(A)**

RATIONALE

9.22   SA is a major cause of morbidity in dialysis patients. It is the commonest cause of HD access related sepsis and the second commonest organism responsible for peritonitis in PD patients. Most infections arise from the patient's own flora and there is now a strong link between nasal carriage of SA and the risk of subsequent clinically important infection.[14] The carriage of MRSA has further implications. MRSA is usually resistant to multiple antibiotics and individuals who develop MRSA infections may well not respond to the initial antibiotic selected before culture results are available. Both attributable death rate and length of hospitalisation are higher in those infected with MRSA compared with fully sensitive SA.[15] There is also the potential for transmission to other patient groups within the hospital, passing on the associated risks as well as contributing to hospital colonisation. Development of further antibiotic resistance is also a concern. First line use of antibiotics such as vancomycin has been associated with the development of intermediate resistance to these agents.[16] If these new strains become widespread then the consequences may be devastating.

9.23   A coherent infection control policy involves everyone associated with the care of renal patients and needs to be constructed in consultation with interested parties and then widely disseminated. All aspects of access management should be examined.

Protocols for the creation and maintenance of HD access and PD catheters should be followed and guidance established for intervention when problems arise. The incidence of SA nasal carriage in dialysis populations is around 50%, with MRSA rates usually reflecting endemic levels in the local hospital.[17] To monitor the problem, screening is required. Around 80% of SA carriers will be identified from a single nasal swab, which offers the most cost effective and convenient method of detection.[18] Topical treatment with 2% mupirocin cream is currently the most reliable method of clearing nasal colonisation. It is effective against both SA and MRSA although recolonisation can be detected in 50% by four months.[19,20] This would suggest that if intervention protocols are planned then screening is required on a regular basis; three-monthly would seem reasonable.

9.24   Patients with temporary central venous dialysis catheters are at particular risk of line-related SA infections. Two separate prospective randomised studies have examined the efficacy of applying anti-microbial agents to the catheter exit site. Both 10% povidone-iodine ointment[21] and 2% mupirocin ointment[22] afforded considerable protection against SA exit-site infection, line colonisation and septicaemia (relative risk reduction for septicaemia was 11.5 ($p<0.01$) with 10% povidone-iodine and 7.2 ($p=0.001$) with mupirocin). There are no specific data on effectiveness with tunneled or implantable dialysis lines. Elimination of SA nasal carriage in mixed HD populations using nasal mupirocin cream, has also been studied. Given the high recolonisation rates, most intervention studies have used schedules combining eradication and maintenance treatment. A number of these have demonstrated a significant and substantial reduction in the risk of SA sepsis although the development of mupirocin resistance is a concern and has been documented.[23,24] In an effort to avoid long mupirocin use, a strategy of three-monthly screening and eradication may well be preferable.

9.25   SA exit-site infections and peritonitis are significantly higher in PD patients who are SA nasal carriers. Two prospective studies with historical controls have demonstrated 3–4 fold reduction in SA peritonitis rates by the application of 2% mupirocin ointment to the PD catheter exit site either daily or thrice weekly.[25,26] Oral rifampicin was also shown to be effective although side effects were relatively common.[25] Clearance of nasal SA carriage has also been examined. A prospective randomised trial of regular monthly five-day courses of nasal mupirocin in SA nasal carriers led to a three-fold reduction in SA exit-site infection, although peritonitis rates were not reduced.[27] No evidence of mupirocin resistance was identified but it remains a concern.

9.26   Transmission of SA and MRSA from patient to patient is mainly due to hand contamination. The single most important infection control measure is that of simple hand washing.[28] At all levels the renal unit must develop a culture of regular hand washing or decontamination between patient contacts. Isolation of MRSA-positive patients is also of value in limiting spread particularly during epidemics. In many hospitals this would require further development, including increased provision of single rooms.

References

1 Department of Health. *Rosenheim Report*. London: HMSO, 1972.

2 Alter HJ. The cloning and clinical implications of HGV and HGBV-C. *N Engl J Med* 1996;**334**:1536–7.

3 Masuko K, Matsui T, Iwano K *et al*. Infection with hepatitis GB virus C in patients on maintenance hemodialysis. *N Engl J Med* 1996;**334**:1485–90.

4 Schlaak JF, Köhler H, Gerken G. Hepatitis G virus: an old but newly discovered hepatotropic virus: is it of interest to the nephrologist? *Nephrol Dial Transplant* 1996;**11**:1522–3.

5 Jibani MM, Heptonstall J, Walker AM *et al*. Hepatitis immunization in UK renal units: failure to put policy into practice. *Nephrol Dial Transplant* 1994;**9**:1765–8.

6 Department of Health/Health and Safety Commission. Advisory Committee on Dangerous Pathogens. *Protection against blood-borne infections in the workplace; HIV and hepatitis*. London: HMSO, 1995.

7 Expert Advisory Group on AIDS and the Advisory Group on Hepatitis. *Guidance for clinical health care workers: protection against infection with blood-borne viruses; recommendations of the Expert Advisory Group on AIDS and the Advisory Group on Hepatitis*. London: DH, 1998.

8 Advisory Committee on Microbiological Safety of Blood and Tissues for Transplantation. *Guidance on the microbiological safety of human tissues, organs and cells used in transplantation*. London: DH, 2000.

9 Köhler H, Arnold W, Renschin G *et al*. Active hepatitis B vaccination of dialysis patients and medical staff. *Kidney Int* 1984;**25**:124–8.

10 Sampietro M, Badalamenti S, Graziani G. Nosocomial hepatitis C in dialysis units. *Nephron* 1996;**74**: 251–60.

11 Allender T, Medin C, Jacobson SH *et al*. Hepititis C transmission in a hemodialysis unit: molecular evidence for spread of virus among patients not sharing equipment. *J Med Virol* 1994;**43**:415–19.

12 Simon N, Courouce M, Lemarrec N *et al*. A twelve-year natural history of hepatitis C virus infection in hemodialyzed patients. *Kidney Int* 1994;**46**:504–11.

13 Department of Health. *Transmissible spongiform encephalopathy agents: safe working and the prevention of infection*. London: DH, 1998.

14 von Eiff C, Becker K, Machka K *et al*. Nasal carriage as a source of *Staphylococcus aureus* bacteremia. Study Group. *N Engl J Med* 2001;**344**(1):11-16.

15 Rubin RJ, Harrington CA, Poon A *et al*. The economic impact of *Staphylococcus aureus* infection in New York City hospitals. *Emerg Infect Dis* 1999;**5**(1):9-17.

16 Smith TL, Pearson ML, Wilcox KR *et al*. Emergence of vancomycin resistance in *Staphylococcus aureus*. Glycopeptide-Intermediate *Staphylococcus aureus* Working Group. *N Engl J Med* 1999;**340**(7):493–501.

17 Kluytmans J, van Belkum A, Verbrugh H. Nasal carriage of *Staphylococcus aureus*: epidemiology, underlying mechanisms, and associated risks. *Clin Microbiol Rev* 1997;**10**(3):505–20.

18 Coello R, Jimenez J, Garcia M *et al*. Prospective study of infection, colonization and carriage of methicillin-resistant *Staphylococcus aureus* in an outbreak affecting 990 patients. *Eur J Clin Microbiol Infect Dis* 1994;**13**(1):74–81.

19 Bommer J, Vergetis W, Andrassy K *et al*. Elimination of *Staphylococcus aureus* in hemodialysis patients. *ASAIO J* 1995;**41**(1):127–31.

20 Harbarth S, Dharan S, Liassine N *et al*. Randomized, placebo-controlled, double-blind trial to evaluate the efficacy of mupirocin for eradicating carriage of methicillin-resistant *Staphylococcus aureus*. *Antimicrob Agents Chemother* 1999;**43**(6):1412-6.

21 Fong IW. Prevention of haemodialysis and peritoneal dialysis catheter related infection by topical povidone-iodine. *Postgrad Med J* 1993;**69**(Suppl 3):S15-7.

22 Sesso R, Barbosa D, Leme IL *et al*. *Staphylococcus aureus* prophylaxis in hemodialysis patients using central venous catheter: effect of mupirocin ointment. *J Am Soc Nephrol* 1998;**9**(6):1085–92.

23 Boelaert JR, De Smedt RA, De Baere YA *et al*. The influence of calcium mupirocin nasal ointment on the incidence of *Staphylococcus aureus* infections in haemodialysis patients. *Nephrol Dial Transplant* 1989;**4**(4):278–81.

24 Kluytmans JA, Manders MJ, van Bommel E, Verbrugh H. Elimination of nasal carriage of *Staphylococcus aureus* in hemodialysis patients. *Infect Control Hosp Epidemiol* 1996;**17**(12):793–7.

25 Bernardini J, Piraino B, Holley J *et al*. A randomized trial of *Staphylococcus aureus* prophylaxis in peritoneal dialysis patients: mupirocin calcium ointment 2% applied to the exit site versus cyclic oral rifampin. *Am J Kidney Dis* 1996;**27**(5):695–700.

26 Thodis E, Bhaskaran S, Pasadakis P *et al*. Decrease in *Staphylococcus aureus* exit-site infections and peritonitis in CAPD patients by local application of mupirocin ointment at the catheter exit site. *Perit Dial Int* 1998;**18**(3):261–70.

27 Nasal mupirocin prevents *Staphylococcus aureus* exit-site infection during peritoneal dialysis. Mupirocin Study Group. *J Am Soc Nephrol* 1996;**7**(11):2403–8.

28 Solberg CO. Spread of *Staphylococcus aureus* in hospitals: causes and prevention. *Scand J Infect Dis* 2000;**32**(6):587–95.

10 The management of patients approaching end stage renal disease

10.1 Patients with renal failure frequently die prematurely from cardiovascular disease. The rate of decline of renal function can be influenced by a variety of interventions. Thus the objectives of the management of chronic renal failure are to slow the rate of decline of renal failure, and to prolong survival, as well as to treat the effects of this condition and prevent complications. Additional important goals are minimising symptoms and reducing psychosocial morbidity.

Recommendation

▶ Patients with progressive renal failure should be managed in a clinic with multidisciplinary support from dieticians and specialist nurses. (**Good practice**)

RATIONALE

10.2 Progressive renal failure results in the retention of nitrogenous waste products and metabolic and endocrine dysfunction. The key elements of care include:

▷ blood pressure management

▷ correction of anaemia (see Chapter 7)

▷ prevention of disordered calcium/phosphate metabolism

▷ control of acidosis, and

▷ education and preparation for dialysis including vascular access (see Chapter 3).[1,2]

In addition, needling forearm veins should be avoided so that they may be used for vascular access. It is important that patients with diabetes have good glucose control and that there is liaison between diabetic and renal services.

10.3 Patients are not only at risk of developing sodium retention, hyperphosphataemia, and hyperlipidaemia, but also tend to reduce their protein intake spontaneously as uraemia progresses.[3] Patients benefit from dietary advice from dieticians trained in the dietary management of renal disease.

10.4 Patients need information and advice about end stage renal disease (ESRD), and the impact this will have on their lifestyle, in order to make an informed decision about whether to accept dialysis treatment, and about which modality would suit them best. Patients need access to clinicians, nurses and social workers to obtain such information and are therefore best managed in a setting where all these professionals are available on a single clinic visit. This may be achieved most easily in a dedicated pre-dialysis clinic.

▶ Blood pressure targets are 125/75 mmHg for those with progressive proteinuric renal disease and 130/80 mmHg for those with stable renal function. **(A)**

▶ Angiotensin converting enzyme (ACE) inhibitors should be considered as the agents of first choice in the management of hypertension in patients with progressive renal disease. **(A)**

Recommendations

▶ Patients should be advised where necessary to stop smoking. **(B)**

▶ Patients should be advised where necessary to reduce dietary salt intake, take regular exercise, and reduce alcohol intake. **(C)**

RATIONALE

10.5   The cardiovascular mortality of patients on the ESRD programmes is much greater than that of the general age-matched population (Chapter 6).[4] Although this may reflect changes secondary to uraemia, good blood pressure control at an early stage of their illness could potentially reduce the subsequent prevalence of cardiovascular disease in the dialysis population. Hypertension is also a major risk factor for the progression of renal disease, and exacerbates proteinuria, which itself is an additional risk factor for progression. Several randomised controlled trials have shown that good blood pressure control reduces the rate of progression of both diabetic and non-diabetic renal disease and these have been incorporated into guidelines for the management of hypertension.[5,6]

10.6   Lifestyle changes have a moderate effect in mild to moderate hypertension in the normal population. In patients with progressive renal disease, an increased dietary sodium intake accelerates the decline in renal function, and increases proteinuria.[7] Cigarette smoking is associated with an increase of cardiovascular risk in the general population and with more rapid progression of renal failure.[8–10]

10.7   ACE inhibitors are more effective than other anti-hypertensive agents in slowing the rate of progression of both diabetic and non-diabetic proteinuric renal disease.[11–14] ACE inhibitors are also beneficial after myocardial infarction, and are of primary benefit in high risk groups, such as those with diabetes mellitus or reduced left ventricular ejection fraction.[15,16] The observed risk reduction is greater than that expected from blood pressure control alone. ACE inhibitors therefore should be the first line agents for treating hypertension in patients with impaired renal function, unless there is a contraindication, or another medical condition for which another anti-hypertensive agent is indicated.

10.8   Studies of angiotensin-2 receptor antagonists (A2RAs) suggest that they may also have a cardioprotective effect and a beneficial effect in slowing the rate of progression of renal failure in patients with Type 2 diabetes.[17,18] Patients intolerant of ACE inhibitors should therefore be treated with an A2RA.

10.9   ACE inhibitors are not particularly effective in controlling systolic hypertension, so additional agents may be necessary for optimal blood pressure control. Patients with chronic renal failure (CRF) have increased sympathetic nervous activity, and, unless there are contraindications, β-blockers may be added. Loop diuretics are of benefit if there is evidence of fluid overload. Alpha-blockers and long-acting calcium channel blockers can also be added, as many patients will require multiple agents for optimal blood pressure control. Short-acting dihydropyridine calcium channel blockers should be avoided.

10.10   Several randomised controlled trials have shown that the rate of progression of renal disease in both diabetic and non-diabetic patients was reduced in those achieving lower than target blood pressure.[16] It is possible that even lower diastolic blood pressures than those recommended above may confer additional benefit.[19,20] The Hypertension Optimal Treatment (HOT) study did not show an increase in adverse events in those with the lowest blood pressures.[21]

10.11   Many patients with renal failure are elderly, and the question arises as to whether a different target should be set for them. Several trials have been conducted in older patients (70–84 years), although the number of patients aged 80 or over was too small to analyse. Such patients were shown to benefit from a reduction in the systolic blood pressure to 160 mmHg or less, with a reduction in the incidence of vascular disease.[22] As there are no controlled trial data for older patients with progressive renal disease, the target recommended could be the lowest blood pressure the patient can tolerate without symptomatic hypotension, and 24-hour blood pressure monitoring may be undertaken to exclude asymptomatic episodes.

Nutritional management

Recommendations

▶ Patients should be advised where necessary to lose weight, reduce dietary salt intake, and take regular exercise. (**Good practice**)

▶ Dietary protein intake should be approximately 0.75 g/kg/day. (**B**)

▶ Patients should be regularly screened for undernutrition. (**Good practice**)

▶ Serum bicarbonate should be in the normal range. (**C**)

▶ Serum phosphate should be <1.9 mmol/l. (**B**)

RATIONALE

10.12   Low protein diets reduce the generation of nitrogenous waste products, organic and inorganic acids. The accumulation of some of these waste products of metabolism results in the clinical and metabolic disturbances associated with uraemia. Low protein diets reduce the symptoms of uraemia, but put the patient at risk of malnutrition.[23]

10.13   Several studies designed in the 1980s and early 1990s reported that protein restricted diets could delay progression to ESRD.[24–31] These trials were performed in an era when the importance of very tight blood pressure control was not understood, and without the availability of current potent anti-hypertensive agents.[32,33] A more recent multi-centre

US study found that blood pressure control rather than dietary intervention had an effect on reducing the rate of decline in renal function.[34–37]

10.14   The majority of patients with chronic progressive renal failure spontaneously restrict their protein intake to 0.6–0.7 g/kg/day,[38] and therefore in clinical practice many units do not formally advise restriction of protein intake. Most patients start to reduce both their protein and energy intake once the clearance falls below 50 ml/min.[38] Without professional dietary advice, the majority of patients develop a negative nitrogen balance, due to a combination of inadequate first class protein and calorie intake. It is therefore important that patients are carefully monitored and reviewed by a renal dietician to ensure that they maintain their nutritional status. In general patients are more likely to comply with diets containing at least 0.75 g/kg/day of protein.[32] To prevent malnutrition diets should contain an increased proportion of first class protein, and also an increased calorie content, of up to 35 kcal/kg/day.[39]

10.15   The initiation of dialysis must not be delayed if the patient is becoming malnourished: a low serum urea and creatinine may reflect malnutrition rather than an acceptable glomerular filtration rate (GFR). Serum urea and creatinine not only depend upon renal function, but are also markers of dietary protein intake, muscle bulk and turnover, and physical activity. Thus patients with CRF should be reviewed regularly, and examined for signs of malnutrition.[40] Nutritional screening should be performed regularly, including as a minimum the measurement of height and weight. Body mass index (BMI) and any unintentional loss of oedema free body weight should be recorded. Undernutrition should be considered if the patient has a BMI of <18.5 and/or 10% or greater unintentional loss of oedema free weight in the preceding six months. Several studies have also used the subjective global assessment (SGA) to screen for undernutrition, either as the full score, with detailed anthropometric assessment of the patient, or as a modified score, based on clinical assessment.[41]

10.16   Metabolic acidosis develops with the progression of renal disease, and results in both increased protein catabolism and reduced nutritional intake, thus exacerbating the risk of undernutrition.[42,43] Acidosis also increases the risk of secondary hyperparathyroidism.[44,45] Bicarbonate supplementation can be used to correct metabolic acidosis and improve nutritional state.[42]

10.17   Phosphate retention develops with progressive renal failure and contributes to the development of hyperparathyroidism.[46] Patients need dietetic advice to restrict dietary phosphate without compromising adequate protein intake. Most patients will require phosphate binders to achieve adequate phosphate control. Calcium-based phosphate binders are currently the agents of first choice, but trials of sevalemer may show it to have beneficial effects on vascular calcification when compared with calcium-based binders. Data do not justify it yet as a first-line agent.

10.18   Hyperparathyroidism develops with declining renal function. Oral alfacalcidol or calcitriol can be given to pre-dialysis patients to control or prevent secondary hyperparathyroidism, without causing a deterioration in renal function.[46,47] Such therapy needs to be carefully monitored to prevent the development of iatrogenic hypercalcaemia.

10.19   Initiation of dialysis should be considered in cases of deteriorating nutritional status with no response to dietary modification, and without another underlying cause, as the mortality of patients with undernutrition at the initiation of dialysis is significantly increased.[48,49]

Initiation of dialysis 10.20   Patients reach the need for dialysis by three main routes:

1   by presenting as an acute uraemic emergency, when dialysis is mandatory, and planning impossible;

2   with predictably progressive renal failure – such as polycystic disease or glomerulonephritis; or

3   with a background of relatively stable renal impairment which progresses very slowly – such as post-obstructive atrophy or some cases of renal ischaemia.

The timing of the initiation of dialysis is irrelevant for the first group of patients. Dialysis can be planned and then started early in the second group of patients without undue economic impact. The third group of patients may survive long periods with stable renal function.

Recommendations

▶ Dialysis should be considered when the weekly urea clearance falls below the equivalent of a *Kt/V* of 2.0 (equivalent to a GFR of approximately 14 ml/min). Dialysis will be indicated in such patients if there is evidence of malnutrition or if symptoms interfere with quality of life. It is prudent to consider dialysis at this early stage in those with predictably steadily progressive renal failure as occurs in polycystic disease or glomerulonephritis. Those with relatively stable renal function, however, may often be treated conservatively. (**Good practice**)

▶ All patients should be able to start dialysis when clinically indicated; there should be no waiting list for dialysis. (**Good practice**)

▶ Patients with progressive renal failure should be referred to a nephrologist early in the course of their disease (serum creatinine 150–200 µmol/l) to enable dialysis to be started in a planned fashion. (**Good practice**)

RATIONALE

10.21   Bonomini *et al* reported that early commencement of dialysis, at a GFR in excess of 10 ml/min, was associated with increased survival on dialysis when compared either with historical controls who had started dialysis only when they developed symptoms, or with patients who had commenced dialysis as an emergency.[50–57] Because lead-time bias and case-mix differences were ignored, a causal relationship cannot be inferred. An attempt was made to undertake a cost-effectiveness analysis, but again case-mix biases were ignored.[53] Ratcliffe *et al*[58] also reported an association between poor outcomes and late referral but they included in the 'late referral group' patients who presented late to the medical services and hence could not have been referred earlier. Other authors made similar analyses and conclusions, without adding to our understanding of when to start dialysis.[59–65]

10.22   Kjellstrand et al[66] analysed European and American data and showed that 90% of the variation in mortality in patients on dialysis reflected comorbidity. He could find no major beneficial effect of early commencement of dialysis.

10.23   Churchill[67] reviewed the evidence addressing the optimal time to commence dialysis. He concluded that dialysis should be initiated at a creatinine clearance of 9–14 ml/min if there is evidence of malnutrition.

10.24   The Peritoneal Dialysis Adequacy Work Group of the National Kidney Foundation Dialysis Outcomes Quality Initiative (DOQI)[68] recommended initiation of dialysis when the weekly Kt/V falls below 2.0 unless weight is stable, protein intake is adequate and there are no symptoms attributable to uraemia. In other words, dialysis should be started for clinical rather than purely biochemical reasons.

10.25   At the 2001 UK Renal Association meeting, Traynor and colleagues presented data on 275 patients who had been followed prospectively from a clearance of at least 20 ml/min in order to assess the impact of early dialysis. Survival from this clearance to death was compared between early starters (creatinine clearance >8.3 ml/min) and late starters (<8.3 ml/min). Survival was superior in late starters when assessed from a clearance of 20 ml/min. This suggests that longer survival after dialysis in early starters is at least in part due to lead-time bias. Similarly, the Netherlands Cooperative Study on the Adequacy of Dialysis (NECOSAD) group recently showed that improved survival in those starting dialysis 'early' was accounted for by lead-time bias.[69]

10.26   United States Renal Data System (USRDS) data on all patients commencing dialysis have been analysed with respect to the relationship between starting serum creatinine concentration and survival on dialysis.[70] The relative risk of mortality on dialysis rose sharply as the serum creatinine at the start of dialysis fell. The relative risk of death was 1.71 in those with a serum creatinine of <4 mg/dl (<352 µmol/l) at start of dialysis, 1.58 with creatinine 4–7.9 mg/dl (350–700 µmol/l) and 1.2 with creatinine 8–9.9 mg/dl (700–880 µmol/l). On the other hand, those with a serum creatinine >18 mg/dl (>1584 µmol/l) had a mortality equal to those starting either with a creatinine of 10–11.9 mg/dl (880–1050 µmol/l) or 12–17.9 mg/dl (1050–1580 µmol/l).

10.27   Fink et al made a further analysis of USRDS data.[71] Raw creatinine values at the commencement of dialysis were converted to estimated creatinine clearances using the Modification of Diet in Renal Disease (MDRD) formula. Patients were analysed by quintiles of creatinine clearance at commencement of dialysis, and there was a highly significant inverse correlation between clearance and survival. Mean survival was 827.5 days in the highest clearance quintile compared with 1048.8 days in the lowest clearance quintile.

10.28   A randomised trial of early dialysis has not been undertaken. Such a study, given the controversy discussed above, would be appropriate although there would be many practical difficulties. Potential disadvantages of early dialysis in asymptomatic patients include increased costs, failure of vascular access, increased iatrogenic morbidity, and psychosocial disruption.

10.29   Renal failure is described as progressive when renal function declines over time. This is usually evidenced by a rising serum creatinine. Such patients require interventions to slow the rate of decline of their renal function and to meet the other objectives outlined in 10.1. To this end, they should be referred to a nephrologist when serum creatinine has reached 150–200 µmol/l. The optimal management of individual patients will vary. Some may need to attend a renal clinic regularly and others may be managed by shared care with the patient's general practitioner after initial renal investigation.

Paediatric section

10.30   Care of children with advanced CRF is available in the 13 designated specialist centres in the UK, which provide the full range of multidisciplinary team support.[72] Paediatric care is particularly concerned with the impact of CRF on growth, educational progress, social and psychological functioning.[73]

Indications for initiation of dialysis

Standards

▶ All children should be offered dialysis if their measured or calculated GFR falls to 10–15 ml/min/1.73 m^2 unless the child remains asymptomatic and growth is well maintained. (**Good practice**)

▶ Pre-emptive transplantation should be offered to children in whom the progressive decline in renal function gives sufficient time to prepare them for the transplant list, as transplantation is the goal for all children with ESRD. (**Good practice**)

Recommendation

▶ Paediatric renal units should supply data to the Paediatric Renal Registry, including the time of referral to the paediatric renal unit with growth parameters at that time. Similar indices should be recorded at the time of initiation of dialysis or pre-emptive transplantation. This will provide data for informed discussion about ways of improving late referral and timing of renal replacement therapy (RRT) intervention. (**Good epidemiological practice**)

RATIONALE

10.31   Patients with a GFR of less than 25 ml/min/1.73 m^2 should be under the care of specialised paediatric units. However, the increasing evidence that disturbances in nutritional intakes, bone biochemistry and growth occur early in CRF would suggest the need for those with mild and moderate CRF to have joint paediatric, nephrological and dietetic supervision.[74]

10.32   Indications for initiating RRT in children are based upon a combination of clinical, biochemical and psychosocial assessments which are individualised for each patient. Symptoms such as nausea, vomiting and lethargy are combined with anthropometric data (particularly a fall in height velocity), fluid restriction (especially if compromising adequate nutritional intake), hypertension and biochemical values (residual renal function, hyperkalaemia, hyperphosphataemia, acidosis) to make an evaluation of the need for dialysis. School performance and restricted daily activities are also important factors to consider in children.[75]

10.33 There is no evidence in children that relates nutritional status at the start of dialysis or timing of initiation of dialysis to mortality. Mortality rates are highest in the youngest patients and in particular those with co-morbid features, being as high as 20% in the first two years of life. Thereafter rates fall to approximately 1% per year.[76] There is, however, long-standing evidence that uraemia has a negative impact upon the growth of children, and in turn, a decrease in height of 1 standard deviation score (SDS) is associated with a 14% increase in risk of death.[77] Malnutrition may also contribute to developmental problems, as well as poor growth. Data from UK units would suggest that children commencing RRT are already growth retarded, and this should be a point of particular focus for paediatric nephrologists.[78,79]

Immunisation

Standards

▶ All children should complete a standard course of childhood immunisation as stipulated by the Department of Health (DH).[80] **(C)**

▶ Each unit should have an immunisation policy. It is recommended that hepatitis B, varicella and BCG vaccination after Heaf testing are completed prior to transplantation. **(Good practice)**

Nursing and family support

Standards

▶ All children should be cared for by paediatric nephrology nurses, who deliver specialised care for children who need RRT both in hospital and in the community.[81] **(Good practice)**

▶ Prior to commencing home peritoneal dialysis, a home assessment should be undertaken. **(Good practice)**

▶ All families should have access to other staff who may be involved in the care of the child with CRF, including play staff, schoolteachers, psychologists, psychiatrists and youth workers. **(Good practice)**

Recommendation

▶ All children and families should have access to support from members of the multidisciplinary team. Their information needs should be assessed and met via interviews, booklets, videos and other resources. It is important that phobias, particularly needle phobias, are addressed as these can assume immense importance in the long-term care of a child on RRT.[81] **(Good practice)**

Please refer to the paediatric sections in Chapter 5 for nutritional support and biochemical control, and in Chapter 6 for blood pressure control.

References

1   Petersen JC, Adler S, Burkart JM *et al* (for the Modification of Diet in Renal Disease (MDRD) Study Group). Blood pressure control, proteinuria and the progression of renal disease. *Ann Intern Med* 1995;**123**:754–62.

2   Hunsicker LG, Adler S, Caggiula A *et al* (for the Modification of Diet in Renal Disease (MDRD) Study Group). Predictors of the progression of renal disease in the Modification of Diet in Renal Disease Study. *Kidney Int* 1997;**51**:337–45.

3   Kopple JD. Dietary protein and energy requirements in ESRD patients. *Am J Kidney Dis* 1998; **32**(Suppl 4):S97–104.

4   Foley R, Levey A, Sarnak M. Clinical epidemiology of cardiovascular disease in chronic renal failure. *Am J Kid Dis* 1998;(Suppl 3):S112-9.

5   Guidelines Subcommittee. 1999 World Health Organisation. International Society of hypertension guidelines for the management of hypertension. *J Hypertension* 1999;**17**:151–83.

6   Ramsay LE, Williams B, Johnston DG *et al*. Guidelines for management of hypertension: Report of the Third Working Party of the British Hypertension Society. *J Human Hypertens* 1999;**13**:630–5.

7   Cianciaruso B, Bellizi V, Minutolo R *et al*. Salt intake and renal outcome in patients with progressive renal disease. *Mineral Electr Metab* 1998;**24**:296–301.

8   Bleyer AJ, Shemanski LR, Burke GL *et al*. Tobacco, hypertension and vascular disease: risk factors for renal functional decline in an older populations. *Kidney Int* 2000;**57**:2072–9.

9   Halimi JM, Giraudeau B, Vol S *et al*. Effects of current smoking and smoking discontinuation on renal function and proteinuria in the general population. *Kidney Int* 2000;**58**:1285–92.

10   Stengel B, Couch C, Cenee S, Heman D. Age blood pressure and smoking effects on chronic renal failure in primary glomerular nep. *Kidney Int* 2000;**57**:2519–26.

11   Remuzzi G, Navis G, DeZeeuw D, DeJOng PE. The Gisen Group. Randomised placebo controlled trial of effect of ramipril on decline in glomerular filtration rate and risk of terminal renal failure in proteinuric non-diabetic nephropathy. *Lancet* 1997;**349**:1857–63.

12   Giatras I, Lau J, Levey AS. Effect of angiotensin converting enzyme inhibitors on the progression on non-diabetic renal disease: a meta analysis of randomised trials. *Ann Intern Med* 1997;**127**:337–45.

13   McIntosh A, Hutchinson A, Marshall S *et al*. *Clinical guidelines and evidence review for type 2 diabetes. Renal disease: prevention and management*. London: Royal College of General Practitioners, 2001.

14   Heart Outcomes Prevention Evaluation (HOPE) Study Investigators. Effects of ramipril on cardiovascular and microvascular outcomes in people with diabetes mellitus: results of the HOPE Study and MICRO-HOPE Study. *Lancet* 2000;**355**:253–9.

15   Lewis JB, Beri T, Bain RP *et al* (and the Collaborative Study Group). Effect of intensive blood pressure control on the course of type I diabetic nephropathy. *Am J Kid Dis* 1999;**34**:809–17.

16   Bakris GL. Progression of diabetic nephropathy. A focus on arterial pressure level and methods of reduction. *Diabetes Res Clin Pract* 1998;**39**(supp):S35–42.

17   Lewis EJ, Hunsicker LG, Clarke WR *et al* (for the Collaborative Study Group). Renoprotective effect of the angiotensin-receptor antagonist Irbesartan in patients with nephropathy due to type 2 diabetes. *N Engl J Med* 2001;**345**:851–60.

18   Brenner BM, Cooper ME, de Zeeuw D *et al* (the RENAAL Study Investigators). Effects of Losartin on renal and cardiovascular outcomes in patients with type 2 diabetes and nephropathy. *N Engl J Med* 2001;**345**:861–9.

19   Wight JP, Brown CB, El Nahas AM. Effect of control of hypertension on progressive renal failure. *Clin Nephrol* 1993;**39**:305–11.

20   Toto RD, Mitchell HC, Smith RD *et al*. "Strict" blood pressure control and progression of renal disease in hypertensive nephrosclerosis. *Kidney Int* 1995;**48**:851–9.

21 Hansson L, Zanchetti A, Carruthers SG *et al*. Effects of intensive blood pressure lowering and low dose aspirin in patients with hypertension: Principal results of the Hypertension Optimal Treatment (HOT) Randomised Trial. *Lancet* 1998;**351**:1755–62.

22 MacMahon S, Rogers A. The effects of blood pressure reduction in older patients: an overview of five randomised controlled trials in elderly hypertensives. *J Clin Exp Hypertens* 1993;**15**:967–76.

23 Bergström J. Nutrition and mortality in haemodialysis patients. *J Am Soc Nephrol* 1995;**6**:1329–41.

24 Barsotti G, Giannoni A, Morelli E *et al*. The decline of renal function slowed by very low phosphorus intake in chronic renal failure patients following a low nitrogen diet. *Clin Nephrol* 1984;**21**:54–9.

25 D'Amico G, Gentile MG, Fellin G *et al*. Effect of dietary protein restriction on the progression of renal failure: a prospective randomised trial. *Nephrol Dial Transplant* 1994;**9**:1590–4.

26 Ihle BU, Becker GJ, Whitworth JA *et al*. The effect of protein restriction on the progression of renal insufficiency. *New Engl J Med* 1989;**321**:1773–7.

27 Locatelli F, Alberti D, Graziani G *et al*. Prospective, randomised, multicentre trial of effect of protein restriction on progression of chronic renal insufficiency. The Northern Italian Cooperative Study. *Lancet* 1991;**337**:1299–1304.

28 Locatelli F, Alberti D, Graziani G *et al*. Factors affecting chronic renal failure progression: results from a multicentre trial. The Northern Italian Cooperative Study Group. *Mineral Electrolyte Metabolism* 1992;**295**:295–302.

29 Walser M, Hill SB, Ward L, Madger L. A crossover trial of progression of chronic renal failure: ketoacids versus amino acids. *Kidney Int* 1993;43:933–9.

30 Walser M, Hill S, Ward L. Progression of chronic renal failure on substituting a keto supplement for an amino acid supplement. *J Am Soc Nephrol* 1992;**2**:1178–85.

31 Williams PS, Stevens ME, Fass G *et al*. Failure of dietary protein and phosphate restriction to retard the rate of progression of chronic renal failure: a prospective, randomised, controlled trial. *Q J Med* 1991;**81**:837–55.

32 Kasiske BL, Lakatau JD, Ma JZ, Louis TA. A meta analysis of the effects of dietary protein restriction on the rate of decline in renal function. *Am J Kidney Dis* 1998;**31**:954–61.

33 Pedrini MT, Levey AS, Lau J *et al*. The effect of dietary protein restriction on the progression of diabetic and non-diabetic renal diseases: a meta analysis. *Ann Intern Med* 1996;**124**:627–32.

34 The Modification of Diet in Renal Disease Study Group. Effects of dietary protein restriction on the progression of moderate renal disease in the Modification of Diet Renal Disease Study. *J Am Soc Nephrol* 1996;**7**:2616–26.

35 Klahr S, Andrew S, Levey AS *et al*. The effects of dietary protein restriction and blood pressure control on the progression of chronic renal disease. *N Engl J Med* 1994;**330**:877–84.

36 Levey AS, Adler S, Caggiula AW *et al*. Effects of dietary protein restriction on the progression of advanced renal disease in the Modification of Diet in Renal Disease Study. *Am J Kidney Dis* 1996;**27**:652–3.

37 Levey AS, Greene T, Beck GJ *et al* (for the MDRD Study group). Dietary protein restriction and the progression of chronic renal disease. What have all the results of the MDRD study shown? *J Am Soc Nephrol* 1999;**10**:627–32.

38 Ikizler TA, Greene JH, Wingard RL. Spontaneous dietary protein intake during progression of chronic renal failure. *J Am Soc Nephrol* 1995;**6**:1386–91.

39 Soroka N, Silverberg DS, Greemland M *et al*. Comparison of a vegetable based (soya) and an animal based low protein diet in predialysis chronic renal failure patients. *Nephron* 1998;**79**:173–80.

40 Frisancho AR. New standards of weight and body composition by frame size and height for assessment of nutritional status of adults and the elderly. *Am J Clin Nutr* 1984;**40**:808–19.

41 Detsky AS, McLaughlin JR, Baker JP *et al*. What is subjective global assessment of nutritional status? *J Parent Enteral Nutr* 1987;**11**:8–13.

42 Graham KA, Hoenich NA, Tarbit M *et al*. Correction of acidosis in hemodialysis patients increases the sensitivity of the parathyroid glands to calcium. *J Am Soc Nephrol* 1997;**8**:627–31.

43   Louden JD, Roberts RR, Goodship TH. Acidosis and nutrition. *Kidney Int* 1999 (Suppl);**73**:S85–8.

44   Almaden Y, Hernandez A, Torregrosa V *et al*. High phosphate level directly stimulates parathyroid hormone secretion and synthesis by human parathyroid tissue in vitro. *J Am Soc Nephrol* 1998;**9**:1845–52.

45   Graham KA, Reaich D, Channon SM *et al*. Correction of acidosis in hemodialysis decreases whole-body protein degradation. *J Am Soc Nephrol* 1997;**8**:632–7.

46   Hamdy NA, Kanis JA, Beneton MN *et al*. Effect of alfacalcidol on natural course of renal bone disease in mild to moderate renal failure. *BMJ* 1995;**310**:358–63.

47   Panichi V, Andreini B, De Pietro S *et al*. Calcitriol oral therapy for the prevention of secondary hyperparathyroidism in patients with predialytic renal failure. *Clin Nephrol* 1998;**49**:245–50.

48   Canada-USA (CANUSA) Peritoneal Dialysis Study Group. Adequacy of dialysis and nutrition in continuous peritoneal dialysis: association with clinical outcomes. *J Am Soc Nephrol* 1996;**7**:198–207.

49   USRDS 1992 Annual data report. Comorbid conditions and correlations with mortality risk among 3,399 incident hemodialysis patients. *Am J Kidney Dis* 1992;**20**:32–8.

50   Bonomini V, Vangelista Astefoni S. Early dialysis in renal substitutive programs. *Kidney Int* (Suppl) 1978;**8**:S112–6.

51   Bonomini V. Early dialysis 1979. *Nephron* 1979;**24**:157–60.

52   Bonomini V. Early dialysis up-dated. *Int J Artif Org* 1981;**4**:54–5.

53   Bonomini V, Baldrati L, Stefoni S. Comparative cost/benefit analysis in early and late dialysis. *Nephron* 1983;**33**:1–4.

54   Bonomini V, Feletti C. Early dialysis. *Contrib Nephrol* 1984;**37**:45–51.

55   Bonomini V. Early dialysis stands the test of time. *Life Support Syst* 1985;**3**:1–5.

56   Bonomini V, Feletti C, Scolari MP, Stefoni S. Benefits of early initiation of dialysis. *Kidney Int (Supplement)* 1985;**17**:S57–9.

57   Bonomini V, Feletti C, Vangelista A, Stefoni S. Early dialysis and renal transplantation. *Nephron* 1986;**44**:267–71.

58   Ratcliffe PJ, Phillips RE, Oliver DO. Late referral for maintenance dialysis. *BMJ* 1984;**288**:441–3.

59   Innes A, Rowe PA, Burden RP, Morgan AG. Early deaths on renal replacement therapy: the need for early nephrological referral. *Nephrol Dial Transplant* 1992;**7**:467–71.

60   Jungers P, Zingraff J, Albouze G *et al*. Late referral to maintenance dialysis: detrimental consequences. *Nephrol Dial Transplant* 1993;**8**:1089–93.

61   Jungers P, Zingraff J, Page B *et al*. Detrimental effects of late referral in patients with chronic renal failure: a case-control study. *Kidney Int* (Suppl) 1993;**41**:S170–3.

62   Ifudu O, Dawood M, Homel P, Friedman EA. Excess morbidity in patients starting uremia therapy without prior care by a nephrologist. *Am J Kidney Dis* 1996;**28**:841–5.

63   Sesso R, Belasco AG. Late diagnosis of chronic renal failure and mortality on maintenance dialysis. *Nephrol Dial Transplant* 1996;**11**:2417–20.

64   Ellis PA, Reddy V, Bari N, Cairns HS. Late referral of end-stage renal failure. *Q J Med* 1998;**91**:727–32.

65   Arora P G, Obrador T, Ruthazer R *et al*. Prevalence, predictors, and consequences of late nephrology referral at a tertiary care center. *J Am Soc Nephrol* 1999;**10**:1281–6.

66   Kjellstrand CM, Hylander B, Collins AC. Mortality on dialysis - on the influence of early start, patient characteristics, and transplantation and acceptance rates. *Am J Kidney Dis* 1990;**15**:483–90.

67   Churchill DN. An evidence-based approach to earlier initiation of dialysis. *Am J Kidney Dis* 1997;**30**: 899–906.

68   National Kidney Foundation. DOQI Clinical practice guidelines for peritoneal dialysis adequacy. *Am J Kidney Dis* 1997;**30**(Suppl 2):S70–3.

69 Korevaar JC, Jansen UA, Dekker FW *et al*. When to initiate dialysis: effect of proposed US guidelines on survival. *Lancet* 2001;**358**:1046–50.

70 US Renal Data System (1992). USRDS 1992 Annual Report. Bethesda, MD: The National Institutes of Health, National Institute of Diabetes and Digestive and Kidney Diseases.

71 Fink JC, Burdick RA, Kurth SJ *et al*. Significance of serum creatinine values in new end-stage renal disease patients. *Am J Kidney Dis* 1999;**34**:694–701.

72 Royal College of Nursing. *Paediatric nephrology nursing. Guidance for nurses*. London: RCN, 2000.

73 Warady BA, Alexander SR, Watkins S *et al*. Optimal care of the paediatric end-stage renal disease patient on dialysis. *Am J Kidney Dis* 1999;**33**;567–83.

74 Norman LJ, Coleman JE, MacDoandl IA *et al*. Nutrition and growth in relation to severity of renal disease in children. *Pediatr Nephrol* 2000;**15**:259–65.

75 Fivush BA, Jabs K, Neu AM *et al*. Chronic renal insufficiency in children and adolescents: the 1996 annual report of NAPRTCS. *Pediatr Nephrol* 1998;**12**:328–37.

76 Kari JA, Gonzalez C, Lederman SE *et al*. Outcome and growth of infants with severe chronic renal failure. *Kidney Int* 2000;**57**:1681–7.

77 Wong CS, Gipson DS, Gillen DL *et al*. Anthropometric measures and risk of death in children with end-stage renal disease. *Am J Kidney Dis* 2000;**36**:811–19.

78 Rigden SPA. Chronic renal failure. In: Postlethwaite RJ (ed). *Clinical paediatric nephrology*, 2nd edn. London: Butterworth, 1994;279.

79 Lewis M. *Report of the Paediatric Renal Registry 1999* (*Second Annual Report* of the UK Renal Registry 1999);**15**:175–87. Bristol: UK Renal Registry, 1999.

80 Department of Health. *Immunisation against infectous disease*. London: HMSO.

81 Watson AR. Strategies to support families of children with end-stage renal failure. *Pediatr Nephrol* 1995;**9**:628–31.

11 | Acute renal failure

11.1   Acute renal failure (ARF) is diagnosed when renal excretory function declines over hours or days. It is usually recognised when serum values of urea and creatinine are rising, more or less rapidly. There are many causes: medical, surgical, traumatic, obstructive and obstetric. The prognosis varies with the cause, both for patient survival and recovery of renal function.

11.2   ARF is a common condition; some degree of acute impairment of renal function occurs in about 5% of hospital admissions.[1] Accurate epidemiological data are very sparse, particularly on incidence. A community-based study in 1993 found that 172 per million adults per year developed severe ARF (serum creatinine concentration >500 µmol/l), with 22 per million adults receiving acute dialysis, and it was estimated that an appropriate referral rate for specialised opinion would be 70 per million population per year.[2] ARF was more common with increasing age, the highest incidence being in those aged 80 years or more, but the largest absolute numbers occurring in those aged between 60 and 79 years. A prospective hospital-based study conducted over a period of 11 weeks in mid-2000 in the Grampian, Highland and Tayside Health Board areas, which include two large teaching hospitals, showed the incidence of renal replacement therapy (RRT) for ARF to be 131 per million per year, with a further 72 per million per year receiving this treatment for acute on chronic renal failure.[3]

11.3   There have been substantial changes in the causes of ARF over the last forty years, together with a progressive increase in the age of those referred to renal units, with the median now 60–65 years.[4] The outcome of comparable cases has undoubtedly improved over this period, but crude figures of survival rates in published series have not always demonstrated this, because these improvements have been offset by inclusion of more and more elderly and severely ill patients.

11.4   Two types of ARF should be distinguished:

1   Isolated failure of the kidneys alone, with other organ systems functioning normally, at least to begin with.

2   Multiple organ failure.

Mortality is low in those with renal failure alone (<5%), whereas it is high (>40%) in those with multiple organ failure. Kidney function may or may not recover depending on the cause of the problem. Most patients will have the condition commonly known as acute tubular necrosis. In these, renal function usually recovers if the patient survives the causative insult. However, active treatment of serious medical and surgical problems in older patients, who frequently have impaired pre-morbid renal function and multiple co-morbidities, has revealed many whose kidneys fail to recover such that they require long-term dialysis, or who achieve only partial recovery, though are able to stop dialysis treatment.[5,6] These patients present not only major problems of clinical management and rehabilitation but extra costs which have not yet been accurately defined, although they now account for around 10% of all patients entering long-term renal replacement therapy programs.[5]

11.5 The case-mix in different units treating ARF will vary according to local clinical activity, eg the proportion of patients with ARF in the context of multiple organ failure will all be increased by the presence of a large intensive care unit (ICU), a trauma unit, an oncology or bone marrow transplant unit, or a liver or cardiothoracic surgical service. This issue is critically important when any comparisons are made of the activities and outcomes between units.

Where patients should be managed?

Recommendations

▶ Renal wards admitting patients with ARF require either a designated high dependency unit (HDU) or access to a centralised HDU where, in addition to RRT, the following are available: close nursing supervision, oxygen, continuous electrocardiogram (ECG) and oxygen-saturation monitoring, automated blood pressure (BP) monitoring, and central venous pressure (CVP) monitoring facilities and expertise. There should be provision for dialysis on alternate days for all patients with ARF and for daily dialysis for those who require it. (**Good practice**)

▶ Patients with multiple organ failure and those who are haemodynamically very unstable should be managed on an ICU, and be transferred there in a timely manner. (**Good practice**)

▶ Whilst it is reasonable for patients with uncomplicated ARF to receive dialysis on a chronic dialysis unit, it is bad practice for this to be done without adequate on-site medical supervision. (**Good practice**)

RATIONALE

11.6 The location in which patients are managed raises controversial issues. Comments and recommendations have to be made in the context that in the UK in 1998 the Audit Commission report identified 252 ICUs, of which 61% said that they provided RRT of some sort. In a nationwide study in 1991, only 20% of nearly 2,000 patients with ARF were transferred to a renal centre.[7] It is unlikely that this has altered. ARF affecting only the kidneys varies in severity, but can in most cases be managed in an area with HDU and haemodialysis/haemofiltration facilities. This may be part of the renal ward or in a centralised HDU. In this area the following should be available: close nursing supervision, oxygen, continuous ECG and oxygen-saturation monitoring, automated BP monitoring, and CVP monitoring facilities and expertise. It should be possible to provide dialysis on alternate days, with daily dialysis if indicated, eg for severe hyperkalaemia and hyper-catabolism. Patients with multiple organ failure including renal failure should be managed within an ICU. This will often require transfer of the patient to another hospital which should be carried out in a timely fashion, supervised by an experienced and properly equipped transfer team[8] in accord with the recommendations of the report of the Working Group on Guidelines on Admission to and Discharge from ICUs and HDUs.[9]

11.7 For any patient with ARF, full support services, including access to specialist interpretation of renal biopsies and a variety of imaging techniques, microbiology etc, are needed.

Techniques of treatment and when to start

RATIONALE

11.8 There are no absolute rules as to when treatment for ARF should begin, but it is better to begin treatment too soon, rather than too late. When it is obvious that ARF is established, RRT should be started before complications occur. Indications for immediate treatment include hyperkalaemia (causing significant ECG changes), severe pulmonary oedema, uraemic acidosis (causing cardiac compromise), and gross uraemia. These situations should be avoided, and not allowed to arise in patients under observation in hospital. It is common practice to begin RRT when the serum urea is raised above 30 mmol/l, but this depends also upon the rate of rise and the clinical setting. Serum urea levels greater than 45 mmol/l usually require urgent institution of therapy.

11.9 Patients with ARF who are haemodynamically stable can be managed using a variety of techniques. Regular intermittent haemodialysis (HD) (see Chapter 3) is the commonest mode of management, but peritoneal dialysis (PD) is still used and is adequate for some non-catabolic cases. Bicarbonate dialysate should be used for acute intermittent dialysis of patients with ARF. Requirements for the technical aspects of HD are the same as those for chronic HD (see Chapter 3). The relatively sudden fluid shifts of acute HD are often poorly tolerated by those who are haemodynamically unstable or those with cerebral oedema (eg liver failure or cerebral injury). For these, continuous renal replacement techniques offer clear advantages, although these are still not available on most renal wards on a 24-hour basis. This type of treatment will usually be given as continuous haemofiltration using a veno-venous circuit and a blood pump. Other techniques may be used according to individual needs and local skills, eg pumped continuous HD, pumped continuous haemodiafiltration. Pumpless arteriovenous haemofiltration should no longer be used. Many variations are available, and there is no evidence on which is best.

11.10 For patients with acute renal failure, there have been suggestions that particular technical aspects of dialysis treatment are important, in particular the use of more rather than less biocompatible membranes. A number of randomised controlled trials have been performed. These have drawn conflicting conclusions, but taken overall there is a trend to show a benefit of non-complement activating membranes.[10] There is evidence from one randomised controlled trial of patients with acute renal failure receiving continuous veno-venous haemofiltration to suggest that filtration rates of 35 or 45 ml/hr/kg produce better outcomes than the lower rate of 20 ml/hr/kg.[11] A recent randomised trial that assigned patients with acute renal failure to receive daily or alternate-day intermittent haemodialysis found that daily treatment resulted in better control of uraemia, fewer hypotensive episodes during dialysis and more rapid resolution of acute renal failure.[12]

Access to specialist nephrological services

11.12   Patients with ARF are often extremely ill with multiple problems and can be very difficult to look after. Many cases are looked after in the ICUs of hospitals without a renal specialist. These ICUs should have defined formal links to a local renal centre for advice on the telephone and a visit or visits from a nephrologist. ICUs that treat only a handful of such patients each year should not have to manage them unaided.

Outcome standards, audit measures and clinical governance

11.13   At the moment it is very difficult to set outcome standards for patients with ARF. Despite many attempts,[13,14] no clinical or biochemical index has been developed that can predict individual outcome reliably enough to be useful, though repeated measurements with time may improve prediction.[15] The mortality of those with multiple organ failure is much higher than those with renal failure alone, hence case-mix will have a dominant effect on the outcome for populations treated at one renal unit rather than another. It is, therefore, impossible to stipulate standards that should be achieved by particular units without precise knowledge of case-mix. This information is not available. None of the existing renal registries and few renal units collect systematic data on ARF. Many patients with ARF are managed on ICUs, and half of these in the UK contribute to the Intensive Care National Audit and Research Centre (ICNARC) Case Mix Program database. It would not be possible to collect such data in renal units without substantial financial and logistic support.

11.14   These issues will be increasingly important with the development of clinical governance. The renal community will not be able to make any substantial progress in the management of ARF until mechanisms are developed for collecting detailed information, from all renal units, about the numbers and types of patient being referred, and the treatments that they receive. Referral or consultation on patients with electrolyte problems and acute uraemia, who do not require dialysis, also forms a substantial part of the workload. It is only when adequate data collection methods have been established that it will be possible to define standards that should be achieved by individual renal units, and also to initiate trials that might reveal ways of improving outcome, eg a large multicentre study comparing modified cellulose and synthetic membranes.

Recommendations for research and audit

11.15   Without further information, future editions of this standards and audit document will not be able to base recommendations for the management of patients with ARF on more secure foundation than that possible here. There is a dearth of information. The key requirement is for prospective data collection of case-mix and outcome of all patients receiving a first renal replacement treatment for ARF, perhaps initially within a single region. This would require assessment of severity of acute and chronic ill health of incident patients and might include length of stay in hospital, survival to 30 and 180 days, and recovery of renal function at 30 and 180 days as the main outcome measures. A national comprehensive prospective study of patients receiving RRT for ARF is currently underway in Scotland.

Paediatric section

11.16   The incidence of ARF in children in the UK, based on referral to regional paediatric nephrology units, is estimated to be 7.5 per million population per year[16] and 8 per million population per year in the Yorkshire region.[17] The true incidence is greater as some children with ARF are managed conservatively by general and specialist paediatricians. Unlike adults, the incidence of ARF decreases with age and is highest in the neonatal and infant age group (age-related incidence is 197 per million per year in the Yorkshire region).

Prognosis

11.17   The overall mortality for children with ARF requiring dialysis is approximately 25%, although this varies with age and the cause of renal impairment. For example, the mortality in neonates and infants is 51% after cardiac surgery for congenital heart defects.[17] Pre-renal causes predominate as the cause of ARF for infants and neonates, while intrinsic renal disease such as haemolytic uraemic syndrome (HUS) accounts for the majority of cases in older children. In this latter group the mortality is much lower (3–5%).[15] Although RRT can allow time for successful resolution of intrinsic renal disease, ARF resulting from poor myocardial function following cardiac surgery is usually one element of multi-organ failure as a result of hypoperfusion and hypoxia and is associated with a high mortality. In contrast to adults with ARF, children who survive usually have normal renal function with very few progressing to ESRD.

Recommendations

▶ All children with ARF require discussion with a paediatric nephrologist. Early transfer for investigation and management is essential in those with rapidly deteriorating renal function or in those with haemodynamic or biochemical disturbances. Children with ARF and multi-organ failure require transfer to a designated regional paediatric ICU lead centre. Although most children with ARF recover renal function, nephrological follow-up during childhood is necessary as the long-term prognosis is uncertain. (**Good practice**)

▶ Where children with ARF are provided with dialysis by adult nephrologists for reasons of geography, the child should be primarily under the care of a paediatrician, who will consult when necessary with the regional paediatric unit and discuss complications at an early stage. Transfer to a regional unit is indicated if there is progression to multi-system disease or if it is evident that the child has reached end-stage renal disease. (**Good practice**)

RATIONALE

11.18 Not all children with acute renal impairment require transfer to a paediatric nephrology centre. However, referral is essential in children with evidence of a rapidly declining glomerular filtration rate, as an urgent histological diagnosis may be required to determine if immunosuppressive therapy or plasmapheresis is required. Other indications for referral include oligoanuria complicated by fluid overload, hypertension, hyponatraemia, hyperkalaemia, uncontrolled acidosis or a need for frequent blood transfusion. Although some children with oligoanuria can be managed conservatively,[18] this is best undertaken in a paediatric nephrology unit; early dialysis in this group has the advantage of facilitating nutritional support. Neonates and premature infants with ARF should be treated in a neonatal unit. Infants and children with ARF requiring RRT but without other organ involvement do not usually require admission to a paediatric ICU but should be managed in paediatric nephrology units because of the provision of appropriate medical and nursing expertise and the availability of educational, social and psychological support. Children with ARF complicating multi-organ failure require prompt transfer to a designated regional paediatric ICU lead centre.

11.19 The mode of dialysis is determined by the clinical circumstances, but PD is generally considered the preferred therapy.[19] Haemofiltration and haemodiafiltration are increasing in popularity in paediatric ICU, while HD remains an important mode of RRT which has a role in both paediatric ICU and the renal ward; HD is the preferred mode of treatment in children with renal failure who require plasmapheresis. In major paediatric ICU renal support is increasingly required for children who do not have primary renal disease (eg before and after liver transplantation, oncology patients with tumour lysis and following bone marrow transplantation). In most instances HD is the most appropriate form of RRT. There has been recent publicity regarding the use of haemofiltration in children with meningococcal sepsis but without significant renal impairment; this treatment remains of unproven benefit[20] and its use in paediatric ICUs should be audited.

Recommendations for audit

Recommendation

▶ As for adults, there is no evidence for the optimum level of renal function for starting RRT, or for the optimum dialysis modality. As there is no national database, individual units should collect this data, along with patient outcome. (**Good epidemiological practice**)

References

1   Hou SH, Bushinsky DA, Wish JB *et al*. Hospital-acquired renal insufficiency: a prospective study. *Am J Med* 1983;**74**(2):243–8.

2   Feest TG, Round A, Hamad S *et al*. Incidence of severe acute renal failure in adults: results of a community based study. *BMJ* 1993;**306**(6876):481–3.

3   Metcalfe W, Simpson M, Khan IH *et al*. Acute renal failure requiring renal replacement therapy: incidence and outcomes. *Q J Med* 2002 (in press).

4   Turney JH, Marshall DH, Brownjohn AM *et al*. The evolution of acute renal failure, 1956-1988. *Q J Med* 1990;**74**(273):83–104.

5   Bhandari S, Turney JH. Survivors of acute renal failure who do not recover renal function. *Q J Med* 1996;**89**(6):415–21.

6   Firth JD. Acute irreversible renal failure. *Q J Med* 1996;**89**:397–9.

7   Stevens PE, Rainford DJ. Continuous renal replacement therapy: impact on the management of acute renal failure. *Br J Intensive Care* (Nov-Dec) 1992:361–9 (intermittent pages).

8   Intensive Care Society. *Guidelines for transport of the critically ill adult.* Intensive Care Society, 2002 www.ics.ac.uk. ICS.html

9   Department of Health. *Guidelines on admission to and discharge from intensive care and high dependency units.* London: DH (NHS Executive), 1996.

10 Vanholder R, De Vriese A *et al.* The role of dialyzer biocompatibility in acute renal failure. *Blood Purif* 2000;**18**(1):1–12.

11 Ronco C, Bellomo R, Homel P *et al.* Effects of different doses on continuous veno-venous haemo-filtration on outcomes of acute renal failure: a prospective randomised trial. *Lancet* 2000;**356**:26–30.

12 Schiffe H, Lang SM, Fischer R. Daily hemodialysis and the outcome of acute renal failure. *N Engl J Med* 2002;**346**:305–10.

13 Knaus WA. Organ system dysfunction and risk prediction. *Intensive Care Med* 1993 **19**(3):127–8.

14 Atkinson SD, Bihari *et al.* (1994). Identification of futility in intensive care. *Lancet* 1994;**344**(8931):1203–6.

15 van Bommel EF, Bouvy ND *et al.* Use of APACHE II classification to evaluate outcome and response to therapy in acute renal failure patients in a surgical intensive care unit. *Ren Fail* 1995 **17**(6):731–42.

16 British Association for Paediatric Nephrology. *The provision of services in the UK for children and adolescents with renal disease.* Report of a working party. BAPN, March 1995.

17 Moghal NE, Brocklebank JT, Meadow SR. A review of acute renal failure in children: incidence, etiology and outcome. *Clin Nephrol* 1998;**49**:91–5.

18 Schulman SL, Kaplan BS. Management of patients with hemolytic uremic syndrome demonstrating severe azotemia but not anuria. *Pediatr Nephrol* 1996 Oct;**10**(5):671–4.

19 Ehrich JHH. Acute renal failure in infants and children. *Int J Art Organs* 1996;**19**:121–3.

20 Best C, Walsh J, Sinclair J, Beattie J. Early haemo-diafiltration in meningococcal septicaemia. *Lancet* 1996;**347**(8995):202.

Appendix A

Summary of items for audit

All standards in this document have linked audit items listed here, as have some of the recommendations. Not all items here are currently subject to audit. Audit items may be collected on a national, local, renal unit or on an individual patient basis. Some are already being collected by the UK Renal Registry and some by the UK Transplant Support Service Authority. Others are collected by individual units to audit local practice.

Epidemiological data

▷ Number of patients (per million population per year) accepted for renal replacement therapy (RRT) for end-stage renal disease (ESRD) by Health Authority or Health Board areas (using Renal Registry definition of acceptance) with starting date.

▷ Renal unit registered with, and providing data to, either UK or Scottish Renal Registry.

▷ Patient survival analysed from day 0 (day of starting uninterrupted dialysis) and from day 90.

Haemodialysis for patients with ESRD

▷ Documentation showing that equipment, disposable items, water and water-testing procedures meet standards.

▷ Dialysate buffer used (eg bicarbonate).

▷ Dialysis membrane used (cellulose, modified cellulose, synthetic low flux or synthetic high flux).

▷ MDA Bulletin DB2000(04) *Single use medical devices: implications and consequences of reuse* read by those reusing dialysers.

▷ Number of haemodialysis (HD) sessions per week.

▷ Measure of adequacy (either urea reduction rate (URR) or equilibrated *Kt/V*).

▷ Nature of vascular access for HD and date of creation.

▷ Number of hypotensive episodes on dialysis.

Peritoneal dialysis for patients with ESRD

▷ Availability, in peritoneal dialysis units, of continuous ambulatory peritoneal dialysis (CAPD), automated peritoneal dialysis (APD) and backup HD facilities.

▷ Documentation showing that equipment and disposable items meet standards.

▷ Nature of transfer system (eg disconnect).

▷ Measure of dialysis adequacy.

▷ Measure of peritoneal transport characteristics (PET).

▷ Blood pressure.

▷ Peritonitis rate (by renal unit).

Nutrition and biochemical standards	▶ Serum bicarbonate (immediately before dialysis for HD patients).
	▶ Plasma parathyroid hormone.
	▶ Serum phosphate.
	▶ Serum calcium.
	▶ Serum potassium (immediately before dialysis in HD patients).
	▶ Serum aluminium.
	▶ Nutritional screen performed.
Cardiovascular risk factors	▶ Blood pressure (before and after dialysis session for HD patients).
Anaemia	▶ Haemoglobin.
	▶ Serum ferritin or percentage hypochromic red blood cells.
Transplantation	▶ Number (per million population per year), age, postcode, and ethnic grouping of patients on waiting list.
	▶ Length of time on waiting list for transplant.
	▶ Written acceptance criteria for transplantation available in unit.
	▶ Letters of explanation sent to all patients not on waiting list.
	▶ Annual review of waiting list patients taken place.
	▶ Human major histocompatibility complex (HLA) antibody status noted for each patient on waiting list.
	▶ Number of donor kidneys retrieved (per million population per year).
	▶ Number (per million population per year), age, postcode, and ethnic grouping of patients transplanted (both from living-related and cadaver donors).
	▶ Pre-transplant cross match test result documented.
	▶ Number of patients receiving a favourably matched kidney.
	▶ Written policy on immunosuppressive protocols, cytomegalovirus, pneumocystis and renal vein thrombosis prophylaxis, and management of delayed graft function available in renal unit.
	▶ Plasma creatinine in patients with functioning grafts.
	▶ Recipient blood pressure.
	▶ Kidney transplant survival noted for each patient.
	▶ Patient survival with a kidney transplant noted for each patient.

Blood-borne viruses and microbiology in dialysis and transplant units	▶	Hepatitis B virus (HBV) immunisation status of patients with chronic renal failure (both those approaching and those on dialysis).
	▶	HBsAg status.
	▶	Hepatitis C virus (HCV) and HIV antibody status.
	▶	Location of dialysis for blood borne virus carriers.
	▶	Use of dedicated machines for HBV carriers.
	▶	Staff HBsAg status.
	▶	Presence of documented infection control policy.

} with record of patient's informed consent.

Patients approaching ESRD	▶	Blood pressure.
	▶	Serum bicarbonate.
	▶	Serum phosphate.

Additional data on children

Paediatric HD	▶	Number of children undergoing HD outwith a tertiary referral centre.
	▶	Number of line infections (in children dialysed using central venous lines).
	▶	Availability of psychosocial support.

| **Paediatric peritoneal dialysis** | ▶ | Number of children undergoing peritoneal dialysis without a tertiary referral centre. |

Nutritional and biochemical standards	▶	Height (or length), weight, head circumference.
	▶	Dietary assessment performed.
	▶	Indicator for and dose of growth hormone.

Transplantation	▶	Proportion of patients listed for pre-emptive transplantation who require dialysis prior to transplantation.
	▶	Provision of written information to parents and child where appropriate.
	▶	Growth (height over 3rd centile and height velocity over 25th centile) attendance following transplant.
	▶	Proportion of patients with zero or one episode of acute rejection still receiving daily steroid therapy at 6 months.

Blood-borne viruses and microbiology in dialysis and transplant units	▶	GFR of children starting dialysis.
	▶	Standard childhood immunisation complete.
	▶	Presence of documented immunisation policy in renal unit.
	▶	Home assessment documented.

Appendix B

Renal services described for non-clinicians

This annex gives information on the issues discussed previously in this document, it also provides background information on renal failure, and discusses the services available for its treatment.

Renal diseases

AB.1 Diseases of the kidney are not as common as cardiovascular conditions or cancers but are much more common than some well-known disorders such as multiple sclerosis or muscular dystrophy. Renal conditions account for about 7,000 deaths per annum according to the Registrar General's figures, but these are probably an underestimate since about one third of deaths of patients with renal failure are not recorded as such in mortality statistics. These figures exclude deaths from cancers of the kidney and associated organs of the urinary tract such as bladder and prostate.

AB.2 Over 100 different diseases affect the kidneys. These diseases may present early with features such as pain, the presence of blood or protein in the urine, or peripheral oedema (swelling of the legs), but much renal disease is self-limiting; it occurs and heals with few or no symptoms or sequelae. On the other hand, some kidney diseases start insidiously and progress but are undetected until renal failure develops.

Acute renal failure

AB.3 Renal failure may be acute and reversible. It occurs in previously normal kidneys when their blood supply is compromised by a fall in blood pressure caused by crush injuries, major surgery, failure of the heart's pumping action, loss of blood, salt or water, or when they are damaged by poisons or overwhelming infection. Renal support is then needed for a few days or weeks before renal function returns. However, about half such patients die during the illnesses because of another condition, often the one which caused the renal failure.

Chronic renal failure and end stage renal disease

AB.4 More common is irreversible chronic renal failure (CRF), in which the kidneys are slowly destroyed over months or years. To begin with there is little to see or find, and this means that many patients present for medical help very late in their disease, or even in the terminal stages. Tiredness, anaemia, a feeling of being 'run down' are often the only symptoms. However, if high blood pressure develops, as often happens when the kidneys fail, or is the prime cause of the kidney disease, it may cause headache, breathlessness and perhaps angina. Ankle swelling may occur if there is a considerable loss of protein in the urine.

AB.5 Progressive loss of kidney function is also called CRF. Early CRF is sometimes referred to as chronic renal impairment or insufficiency, and end stage renal disease (ESRD) when it reaches its terminal stage. At this point, if nothing is done, the patient will die. Two complementary forms of treatment – dialysis and renal transplantation – are available and both are needed if ESRD is to be treated.

AB.6   The incidence of CRF and ESRD rises steeply with advancing age. Consequently an increasing proportion of patients treated for ESRD in this country are elderly and the proportion is even higher in some other developed countries. Evidence from the USA suggests that the relative risk of end stage renal failure in the black population (predominantly of African origin) is 2 to 4 times higher than for whites. Data collected during the review of renal specialist services in London suggest that in the Thames regions there is a similarly greater risk of renal failure in certain ethnic populations (Asian and Afro-Caribbean) than in whites. This is supported by national mortality statistics. People from the Indian subcontinent have a higher prevalence of non-insulin dependent diabetes, and those with diabetes are more likely than whites to develop renal failure. This partly explains the higher acceptance rate of Asians on to renal replacement programmes.

Causes of renal failure

AB.7   Most renal diseases that cause renal failure fall into six categories.

1   Systemic disease. Although many generalised diseases such as systemic lupus, vasculitis, amyloidosis and myelomatosis can cause kidney failure, by far the most important cause is diabetes mellitus (which causes about 20% of all renal disease in many countries). Progressive kidney damage may begin after some years of diabetes, particularly if the blood sugar and high blood pressure have been poorly controlled. Careful lifelong supervision of diabetes has a major impact in preventing kidney damage.

2   Autoimmune disease. 'Glomerulonephritis' or 'nephritis' describes a group of diseases in which the glomeruli (the filters that start the process of urine formation) are damaged by the body's immunological response to tissue changes or infections elsewhere. Together, all forms of nephritis account for about 30% of renal failure in Britain. The most severe forms are therefore treated with medications that suppress response, but treatment makes only a small impact on the progress of this group of patients to end stage renal failure.

3   High blood pressure. Severe ('accelerated') hypertension damages the kidneys, but the damage can be halted – and to some extent reversed – by early detection and early treatment of high blood pressure. This is a common cause of renal failure in patients of African origin.

4   Obstruction. Anything that obstructs the free flow of urine can cause back pressure on the kidneys. Much the commonest cause is enlargement of the prostate in elderly men.

5   Infection of the urine. Cystitis is a very common condition, affecting about half of all women at some time in their lives, but it rarely has serious consequences. However, infections of the urine in young children or patients with obstruction, kidney stones or other abnormalities of the urinary tract may result in scarring of the kidney and eventual kidney failure.

6   Genetic disease. One common disease, polycystic kidneys, and many rare inherited disease, which affect the kidneys, account for about 8% of all kidney failure in Britain. Although present at birth, polycystic kidney disease often causes no symptoms until middle age or later. Understanding of its

genetic basis is rapidly advancing and may lead to the development of effective treatment.

Prevention AB.8 Although many diseases causing CRF cannot be prevented or arrested at present, better control of diabetes and high blood pressure and relief of obstruction have much to offer, provided they are employed early in the course of the disease before much renal damage has occurred. It has also been shown that a group of antihypertensives called angiotension1 converting enzyme inhibitors (ACE1) delay the progression of renal failure. Screening for renal disease has not been .widely practised, because the relatively low incidence of cases renders population screening inefficient and costly. Urine tests for protein or blood, or blood tests for the level of some substances normally excreted by the kidney such as creatinine and urea, are potentially useful methods for screening, if populations at risk for renal failure can be identified, eg diabetics and the elderly.

Complications and comorbidity AB.9 Renal failure is often accompanied by other disease processes. Some are due to the primary disease, eg diabetes may cause blindness and diseases of the nerves and blood vessels. Others, such as anaemia, bone disease and heart failure, are consequences of the renal failure. Coincidental disease such as chronic bronchitis and arthritis are particularly common in older patients with renal failure. In addition many patients with ESRD have diseases affecting the heart and blood vessels (vascular) particularly ischaemic heart disease and peripheral vascular disease. All these conditions, collectively called comorbidity, can influence the choice of treatment for renal failure and may reduce its benefits. Expert assessment of the patient before end stage renal failure can reduce comorbidity and increase the benefit and cost effectiveness of treatment. Thus early detection and referral of patients at risk of renal failure is important.

Renal replacement therapy AB.10 The term renal replacement therapy (RRT) is used to describe treatments for end stage renal failure in which, in the absence of kidney function, the removal of waste products from the body is achieved by dialysis and other kidney functions are supplemented by drugs. The term also covers the complete replacement of all kidney functions by transplantation.

Therapeutic dialysis ('renal dialysis') AB.11 Dialysis involves the removal of waste products from the blood by allowing these products to diffuse across a thin membrane into dialysis fluid which is then discarded along with the toxic waste products. The fluid is chemically composed to draw or 'attract' excess salts and water from the blood to cross the membrane, without the blood itself being in contact with the fluid.

Haemodialysis AB.12 The method first used to achieve dialysis was the artificial kidney, or haemodialysis. This involves the attachment of the patient's circulation to a machine through which fluid is passed, and exchange can take place. A disadvantage of this method is that some form of permanent access to the circulation must be produced to be used at every treatment. Each sessions lasts 4–5 hours and is needed three times a week.

Peritoneal dialysis AB.13 The alternative is peritoneal dialysis, often carried out in the form of continuous ambulatory peritoneal dialysis (CAPD). In this technique, fluid is introduced into the peritoneal cavity (which lies around the bowel) for approximately six hours before withdrawal. The washing fluid must be sterile in order to avoid peritonitis (infection and inflammation of the peritoneum), which is the main complication of the treatment. A silastic tube must be implanted into the peritoneum and this may cause problems such as kinking and malposition. Each fluid exchange lasts 30–40 minutes and is repeated three or four times daily. Neither form of dialysis corrects the loss of the hormones secreted by the normal kidney, so replacement with synthetic erthropoietin and vitamin D is often necessary.

Renal transplantation AB.14 Renal transplantation replaces all the kidneys functions, so erythropoietin and vitamin D supplementation are unnecessary. A single kidney is placed, usually in the pelvis close to the bladder to which the ureter is connected. The kidney is attached to a nearby artery and vein. The immediate problem is the body's acute rejection of the foreign graft, which has largely been overcome during the first months using drugs such as steroids and cyclosporin. These drugs, and others that can be used for that purpose, have many undesirable side effects, including the acceleration of vascular disease. This often means that myocardial infarcts and strokes are commoner in transplant patient than in age-matched controls. During subsequent years there is a steady loss of transplanted kidneys owing to a process of chronic rejection; treatment of this is quite unsatisfactory at the moment, so many patients require a second or even a third graft over several decades, with further periods of dialysis in between.

AB.15 The main problem with expanding the transplantation service is the shortage of suitable kidneys to transplant. Although the situation can be improved it is now clear that, whatever social and medical structures are present and whatever legislation is adopted, there will inevitable be a shortage of kidneys from humans. This remains the case even if kidneys from the newly dead (cadaver kidneys) are retrieved with the maximum efficiency, and living donors (usually, but not always, from close blood relatives of the recipient) are used wherever appropriate. Hope for the future rests with solving the problems of xenotransplantation (which involves using animal kidneys), probably from pigs, although baboons have also been suggested and are closer to humans. Many problems remain unsolved and it is thought highly unlikely that xenotransplantation will become a reliable treatment for end stage renal failure within the next 10 years.

Nature of renal services AB.16 The work of a nephrologist includes the early detection and diagnosis of renal disease and the long-term management of its complications such as high blood pressure, anaemia and bone disease. The nephrologist may share the management with the general practioner or local hospital physician, and relies on them to refer patients early for initial diagnosis and specific treatment. At any one time perhaps only 5% of patients under care are inpatients in wards, the remainder being treated in their homes, another 20% attending the renal unit regularly for haemodialysis. However, inpatient nephrology and the care of patients receiving centre-based dialysis is specialised, complex and requires experienced medical advice to be available on a 24-hour basis. This implies sufficient staff to provide expert cover; cross-covering by inexperienced staff is inappropriate and to be condemned. The other 95% of renal work is sustained on an outpatient basis; this includes RRT by dialysis and the care of transplant patients.

AB.17 There are five major components to renal medicine.

1 RRT. The most significant element of work relates to the preparation of patients in end stage renal failure for RRT and their medical supervision for the remainder of their lives. The patient population will present increasing challenges for renal staffing as more elderly and diabetic patients are accepted for treatment.

2 Emergency work. The emergency work associated with the specialty consists of:

   i Treatment of acute renal failure, often involving multiple organ failure and acute-on-chronic renal failure. Close cooperation with other medical specialties, including intensive care, is therefore a vital component of this aspect of the service.

   ii Management of medical emergencies arising from an end stage renal failure programme. This workload is bound to expand rapidly as the number, age and comorbidity of patients starting RRT increase, and this may interrupt the regular care of patients already on RRT, so increased resources may be required.

3 Routine nephrology. A substantial workload is associated with the immunological and metabolic nature of renal disease which requires investigative procedures in an inpatient setting. It is estimated that 10 inpatient beds per million of the population are required for this work.

4 Investigation and management of fluid and electrolyte disorders. This makes up a variable proportion of the nephrologist's work, depending on the other expertise available in the hospital.

5 Outpatient work. The outpatient work in renal medicine consists of the majority of general nephrology together with clinics attended by dialysis and renal transplant patients.

Further reading   Further details of renal services for renal failure, written for non-physicians, can be found in: Cameron JS. *Kidney failure – the facts*. London: Oxford University Press, 1996.

Appendix C

Glossary

Access
A method of gaining entry to the bloodstream to allow haemodialysis or to the peritoneum for peritoneal dialysis. Access methods used for haemodialysis include a catheter, fistula or graft; a catheter is inserted as peritoneal dialysis access.

Acute renal failure (ARF)
The rapid loss of kidney function over a few hours or days.

Albumin
A type of protein that occurs in the blood.

Alphacalcidol
A form of vitamin D used to treat renal bone disease.

Anaemia
A deficiency of red blood cells which can lead to a lack of oxygen, causing tiredness, shortage of breath and pallor. One of the functions of the kidneys is to produce a hormone epoetin, which helps make blood cells. In kidney failure, epoetin is not made and anaemia results.

Angiotensin converting enzyme inhibitors
Drugs which lower blood pressure, improve heart function and have been shown to delay the progression of renal failure.

Anthropometry
The measuring of the human body or part of the human body.

Antibiotic
A chemical substance produced by a micro-organism which has the capacity, in dilute solutions, to inhibit the growth of or to kill other micro-organisms. Antibiotics are used in the treatment of infectious diseases.

Arteriogram
A type of X-ray that uses a special contrast medium to show the blood vessels. The contrast medium is put into the blood vessels via a tube that is inserted into the groin and passed up to the kidneys.

Artificial kidney
Another name for the dialyser or filtering unit used in haemodialysis.

Atheroma (also called Artherosclerosis)
Deposits of cholesterol and other fats that cause furring and narrowing of the arteries (also called atherosclerosis).

Automated peritoneal dialysis (APD)
A form of peritoneal dialysis that requires a machine to control the movement of fluid into and out of the peritoneal cavity. APD is carried out at home each night whilst the patient sleeps.

Azathioprine
An immuno-suppressant drug used to prevent the rejection of a transplanted kidney.

Beta-blockers
Drugs that slow down the heart rate and lower blood pressure. Examples are atenolol, metoprolol and propranolol.

Bicarbonate
An alkaline substance that is normally present in the blood. A low blood level of bicarbonate shows there is too much acid in the blood.

Biopsy	A test involving the removal of a small piece of an organ or other body tissue and its examination under a microscope.
Bladder	The organ in which urine is stored before being passed from the body.
Blood cells	The microscopically tiny units that form the solid part of the blood. There are three main types: red blood cells, white blood cells and platelets (which are cell fragments).
Blood group	An inherited characteristic of red blood cells. The common classification is based on whether or not a person has A and/or B antigens on their cells. Each person belongs to one of four blood groups. A, B, AB and O.
Blood pressure	The pressure that the blood exerts against the walls of the arteries as it flows through them. Blood pressure measurement consist of two numbers. The first shows the systolic blood pressure, the second, the diastolic blood pressure. The kidneys help to control blood pressure and in kidney failure, the blood pressure tends to be high.
Brain death	A term indicating that the brain has permanently stopped working, and that further life is possible only on a life-support machine. A person must be diagnosed as brain dead before their organs can be removed for a cadaveric transplant.

Cadaveric transplant

A transplant kidney removed from someone who has died.

Calcium	A chemical element obtained through the diet. It is essential for the maintenance of healthy teeth and bone, and is essential for many metabolic processes such as nerve function, muscle contraction and blood clotting.
Catheter	A hollow tube used to transport fluids to and from the body.
Cholesterol	A lipid (sterol) that is a major contributor to atheroma.

Chronic renal failure (CRF)

The slow and progressive deterioration of kidney function. Initially there may be little to see or find, and this means that many patients present for medical help very late in their disease, or even in the terminal stages.

Clearance	The rate at which toxic waste products are removed from the body. Excreting these products is one of the main functions of the kidneys. In kidney failure clearance by the kidneys is inadequate and toxins build up in the blood.
Cochrane Review	A Cochrane Review is a systematic, up-to-date summary of reliable evidence of the benefits and risks of healthcare. Cochrane Reviews are intended to help people make practical decisions. For a review to be called a 'Cochrane Review' it must be in the Parent Database maintained by the Cochrane Collaboration.

Continuous ambulatory peritoneal dialysis (CAPD)

A form of treatment for kidney failure in which fluid is instilled into the patient's peritoneum through a catheter and drained out some hours later. Normally about four such exchanges are performed at regular intervals throughout the day.

Creatinine   A natural waste product of muscle metabolism which is normally excreted by the kidney. When renal function is reduced the level of creatinine in the blood (plasma creatinine) rises and the amount cleared from the kidneys (creatinine clearance) falls..

Creatinine clearance

A calculation to assess the kidneys' ability to remove creatinine from the blood. It is a more accurate guide to how well the kidneys are working than plasma creatinine. Peritoneal creatinine clearance is used as a measure of how well peritoneal dialysis is removing toxins.

Cross-match   The final blood test before a transplant operation is performed. It checks whether the patient has any antibodies to the donor tissue that might damage the transplanted kidney. The operation can proceed only if the cross-match is negative (ie no such antibodies are found).

Cyclosporin   An immunosuppressant drug used to prevent the rejection of a transplant kidney.

Cytomegalovirus (CMV)

A virus that normally causes only a mild 'flu-like' illness. In people with a kidney transplant (and in other people whose immune system is suppressed), CMV can cause a more serious illness, affecting the lungs, liver and blood.

Diabetes Mellitus   A condition in which the blood glucose (sugar) level is higher than normal. It takes two forms: insulin dependent diabetes usually developing in young people and non insulin dependent diabetes seen in these who are elderly or overweight. Both can result in renal failure.

Dialyser   A filtering unit attached to a dialysis machine. It provides the dialysis membrane for patient on haemodialysis. The dialyser removes body wastes and excess water from the blood thus mimicking some of the functions of a normal kidney.

Dialysis   An artificial process by which the toxic waste products of food and excess water are removed from the body while retaining essential substances. Dialysis performs some of the work normally performed by healthy kidneys. It is derived from a Greek word meaning 'to separate'.

Dialysate/Dialysis fluid

A sterile fluid used to remove toxic waste products and water from the body during dialysis.

Dialysis machine   The machine which pumps the patient's blood through the dialyser, and monitors the dialysis process as it takes place. The dialyser or artificial kidney is attached to it.

Dialysis membrane

In haemodialysis a thin layer of cellulose or synthetic fibre with many tiny holes in it, through which the process of dialysis takes place. In peritoneal dialysis, the patient's peritoneum provides the dialysis membrane. In each case, the membrane keeps the dialysis fluid separate from the blood (essential because dialysis fluid is toxic if it flows directly into the blood). The tiny holes in the membrane make it semi-permeable, allowing water and toxic waste substances to pass through and be removed.

Diastolic blood pressure

A blood pressure reading taken when the heart is relaxed. It is taken after the systolic blood pressure and is the second figure in a blood pressure measurement.

Diffusion

A process by which substances pass from a stronger to a weaker solution. Diffusion is one of the key processes in dialysis (the other is ultrafiltration). During dialysis, body wastes such as creatinine pass from the blood into the dialysis fluid. At the same time, useful substances such as calcium pass from the dialysis fluid into the blood.

Donor

A person who donates (gives) an organ to another person (the recipient).

Donor kidney

A kidney that has been donated.

Electrocardiogram (ECG)

A test that shows the electrical activity within the heart.

Echocardiogram (ECHO)

An ultrasound scan showing the structure and function of the heart.

End-stage renal disease (ESRD)

End stage renal disease is reached when chronic renal failure cannot be controlled by conservative management and when the patient requires either dialysis or a kidney transplant in order to maintain life.

End-stage renal failure (ESRF)

An alternative name for end-stage renal disease.

Erythropoietin (Epoetin, epo)

A hormone, made by the kidneys, which stimulates the bone marrow to produce red blood cells.

Exchange

In peritoneal dialysis this term means the process of draining fluid out of the peritoneal cavity and instilling fresh dialysate into the peritoneal cavity.

Exit site

The point where a catheter comes out through the skin. Exit site infections can occur in haemodialysis patients when a catheter is used for access or in those undergoing peritoneal dialysis.

Fistula

A connection between an artery and vein, usually at the wrist or elbow, created surgically to give access to the circulation for haemodialysis. The increased blood flow causes the vein to enlarge, making it suitable for haemodialysis needles.

FK506

Another name for tacrolimus. An immunosuppressant drug used to prevent and treat rejection of a transplanted kidney.

Fluid overload

A condition in which the body contains too much water. It is caused by drinking too much fluid, or not losing enough. Fluid overload occurs in kidney failure because one of the main functions of the kidneys is to remove excess water. Fluid overload is often associated with high blood pressure. Excess fluid first gathers around the ankles (ankle oedema) and may later settle in the lungs resulting in breathlessness (pulmonary oedema).

Glomerulus

One of the tiny filtering units inside the kidney.

Glomerulonephritis (GN)

Inflammation of the glomeruli, which is one of the causes of kidney failure.

Glucose

A type of sugar. There is normally a small amount glucose in the blood. This amount is not usually increased in people with kidney failure unless they also have diabetes mellitus. Glucose is the main solute in peritoneal dialysis fluid, drawing excess water into the dialysis fluid from the blood by osmosis.

Graft

A type of access to the bloodstream for haemodialysis. The graft is a small plastic tube that connects an artery to a vein and is inserted surgically. Haemodialysis needles can then be inserted into the graft. The term graft can also be used for a transplanted kidney.

Haemodialysis (HD)

A form of treatment in which the blood is purified outside the body, by passing it through a filter called the dialyser or artificial kidney. The filter is connected to a machine which pumps the blood through the filter and controls the entire process. For patients with end stage renal disease each dialysis session normally lasts from three to five hours, and sessions are usually needed three times a week.

Haemodialysis catheter

A plastic tube used to gain access to the bloodstream for haemodialysis.

Haemodialysis unit

The part of a hospital where patients go for haemodialysis.

Haemoglobin (Hb) A substance in red blood cells that carries oxygen around the body. Blood levels of haemoglobin are measured to look for anaemia. A low Hb value indicates anaemia.

Heart-beating donor

A term used to describe a donor whose heart is still beating after brain death has occurred. Most, but not all, cadaveric transplants come from heart-beating donors.

Hepatitis

An infection of the liver, usually caused by a virus. Two main types, called hepatitis B and hepatitis C, can be passed on by blood contact. This means that dialysis patients, especially those on haemodialysis, have an increased risk of getting these infections. Care is taken to reduce this risk, and regular virus checks are made on all kidney patients.

Home haemodialysis

Treatment on a dialysis machine installed in a patient's own home.

Hormones

Substances that act as chemical messengers in the body. They are produced in parts of the body called endocrine glands.

Hyperkalaemia

An abnormally high level of potassium in the blood.

Hyperparathyroidism

A disorder in which the parathyroid glands make too much parathyroid hormone.

Immune system

The body's natural defence system. It includes organs such as the spleen and lymph nodes and specialist white blood cells called lymphocytes. The immune system protects the body from infections, foreign bodies and cancer. To prevent rejection of a transplant kidney, it is necessary for patients to take immuno-suppressant drugs.

Immunosuppressant drugs

A group of drugs used to dampen down the immune system to prevent or treat rejection of a transplant kidney. Commonly used examples are cyclosporin, azathioprine and prednisolone. Tacrolimus (FK506), mycophenolate mofetil and rapamycin are newer examples.

Kidneys

The two bean-shaped body organs located at the back of the body, below the ribs. The kidneys remove toxic waste products of protein breakdown and remove excess water from the body. They also help to control blood pressure, manufacture of red blood cells and keep the bones strong and healthy.

Kidney biopsy

Removal of a small piece of kidney through a hollow needle for examination under a microscope. It is required to diagnose some causes of kidney failure; biopsies of transplanted kidneys may also be required.

Kidney donor

A person who gives a kidney for transplantation.

Kidney failure

A condition in which the kidneys are less able than normal to perform their functions of removing toxic wastes, removing excess water, helping to control blood pressure, control red blood cell manufacture and keep the bones strong and healthy. Kidney failure can be acute or chronic. Advanced chronic kidney failure is called end-stage renal disease (ESRD).

Kidney machine

Another name for a dialysis machine.

Kidney transplant

A name both for the transplant operation during which a new kidney is given to a recipient or for the new kidney itself.

Kt/V

A measure of dialysis adequacy.

Lipids

Another name for fats. People with kidney failure tend to have raised lipid levels in the blood.

Living related transplant (LRT)

A transplant kidney donated (given) by a living relative of the recipient. A well-matched living related transplant is likely to function for longer than either a living unrelated transplant or a cadaveric transplant.

Living unrelated transplant

A kidney transplant from a living person who is biologically unrelated to the recipient (such as a husband or wife).

Lymphocytes

Specialist white blood cells that form part of the immune system.

Malnutrition

Loss of body weight, usually due to insufficient intake of foods especially foods providing protein and energy.

Membrane

The material used as a filtering agent in haemodialysers. Many are formed from a cellulose base, others from synthetic materials. The peritoneum is a natural membrane used as the dialysis membrane in peritoneal dialysis.

Methylprednisolone

A drug used to prevent or treat the rejection of a transplant kidney.

Molecule	The smallest unit that a substance can be divided into without causing a change in the chemical nature of the substance.
Nephr-	Prefix meaning 'relating to the kidneys'.
Nephrectomy	An operation to remove a kidney from the body. A bilateral nephrectomy is an operation to remove both kidneys.
Nephritis	A general term for inflammation of the kidneys. Also used as an abbreviation for glomerulonephritis (GN). A kidney biopsy is needed to diagnose nephritis.
Nephrology	The study of the kidneys in health and disease.
Nephrologist	A doctor who cares for patients with kidney disease.
OKT3	Abbreviation for Orthoclone K T-cell receptor 3 antibody, treatment for the rejection of a transplant.
Organ	A part of the body that consists of different types of tissue and that performs a particular function. Examples include kidney, heart and brain.
Osmosis	The process by which water moves from a weaker to a stronger solution through tiny holes in a semi-permeable membrane. In peritoneal dialysis, it is osmosis that causes excess water to pass from the blood into the dialysis fluid.

Parathyroidectomy

An operation to remove the parathyroid glands.

Parathyroid hormone (PTH)

A hormone produced by the parathyroid glands, which helps control blood levels of calcium. When the level of calcium in the blood is low, PTH increases it by causing calcium loss from the bones into the blood.

Peritoneal cavity	The area between the two layers of the peritoneum (or peritoneal membrane) inside the abdomen. The peritoneal cavity contains the abdominal organs, including the stomach, liver and bowels. It normally contains only about 100 ml of liquid, but expands easily to provide a reservoir for the dialysis fluid in peritoneal dialysis.

Peritoneal dialysis (PD)

A treatment of renal failure in which blood purification takes place, using the patient's own peritoneum as the membrane. Bags of dialysis fluid, containing glucose (sugar) and various other substances, are drained in and out of the peritoneal cavity via a PD catheter.

Peritoneal dialysis (PD) catheter

A plastic tube through which dialysis fluid for peritoneal dialysis is drained into, and removed from, the peritoneal cavity. The catheter is about 30 cm (12 in) long and is as wide as a pencil. A small operation is needed to insert the catheter into the abdomen.

Peritoneal equilibration test (PET)

A measurement of the rate at which toxins pass out of the blood into the dialysis fluid during peritoneal dialysis. Patients are described as 'high transporters' (if the toxins move quickly) and 'low transporters' (if the toxins move more slowly). The test is used to assess a patient's suitability for different types of PD.

Peritoneum (peritoneal membrane)

A natural membrane that lines the inside of the wall of the abdomen and that covers all the abdominal organs (the stomach, bowels, liver, etc). The peritoneum provides the dialysis membrane for peritoneal dialysis. It has a large surface area, contains many tiny holes and has a good blood supply.

Peritonitis

Inflammation of the peritoneum which can occur in patients on peritoneal dialysis. It is caused by infecting organisms, usually bacteria and can normally be successfully treated with antibiotics.

Phosphate

A mineral that helps calcium to strengthen the bones. Phosphate is obtained from foods such as diary products, nuts and meat. The kidneys normally help to control the amount of phosphate in the blood. In kidney failure, phosphate tends to build up in the blood.

Phosphate binders

Medication (eg calcium carbonate) that helps prevent a build-up of phosphate in the body. Phosphate binders combine with phosphate in food and the phosphate passes out of the body with the binder.

Potassium

A mineral that is normally present in blood and is removed by the kidney. High values can occur in renal failure which can be dangerous, causing the heart to stop. People with renal failure often need to restrict the amount of potassium in their diet.

Prednisolone

A drug used to prevent the rejection of a transplant kidney.

Radio-isotope scan

A method of obtaining pictures of the body's interior, also called a radionuclide scan. A small amount of a mildly radioactive substance is either swallowed or injected into the bloodstream. The substance gathers in certain parts of the body, which then show up on pictures taken by a special machine.

Radionuclide scan

Another name for a radio-isotope scan.

Randomised Controlled Trial (RCT) (synonym: Randomised Clinical Trial)

An experiment in which investigators randomly allocate eligible people into (eg treatment and control) groups to receive or not to receive one or more interventions that are being compared. The results are assessed by comparing outcomes in the treatment and control groups.

Recipient

In the context of transplantation, a person who receives an organ from another person (the donor).

Red blood cells

Cells in the blood which carry oxygen from the lungs around the body.

Rejection

The process by which a patient's immune system recognises a transplant kidney (or other transplanted organ) as not its 'own' and then tries to destroy it and remove it from the body. Rejection can be acute or chronic.

Renal

Adjective meaning relating to the kidneys.

Renal bone disease

A complication of kidney failure, in which bone abnormalities develop because of low blood levels of calcium and vitamin D and high levels of phosphate. Without treatment, renal bone disease can result in bone pain and fractures.

Renovascular disease

Narrowing of the renal arteries caused by deposite of atheroma ('reno-' means relating to the kidney, and '-vascular' means relating to the blood vessels). Renovascular disease is a common cause of kidney failure in older patients.

Satellite haemodialysis unit

A place where some patients go for haemodialysis away from the main hospital renal unit. They are more suitable for patients whose medical condition is stable, and patients there may do some of the haemodialysis preparation themselves. Such units tend to be more easily accessible to patients than most units in main hospital buildings.

Semi-permeable

An adjective, often used to describe a dialysis membrane, indicating that it will allow some but not all substances to pass through it. Substances made of smaller molecules will pass through the holes in the membrane, whereas substances made of larger molecules will not.

Sphygmomanometer

The instrument used to measure blood pressure.

Staphylococcus

One of a group of bacteria responsible for various infections. It is a common cause of peritonitis in patients on peritoneal dialysis and of catheter infections in haemodialysis patients.

Systolic blood pressure

A blood pressure reading taken when the heart squeezes as it beats. The systolic blood pressure is measured before the diastolic blood pressure and is the first figure in a blood pressure measurement.

Tacrolimus

An immunosuppressant drug used to prevent and treat transplant rejection, also known as FK506.

Tissue type

A set of inherited characteristics on the surface of cells. Each person's tissue type has six components (three from each parent). Although there are only three main sorts of tissue type characteristic (called A, B and DR), each of these exist in several forms. Given the large number of possibilities, it is unusual for there to be an exact tissue type match between a transplant kidney and its recipient. In general, the more characteristics that match, the more likely is a transplant to succeed.

Tissue typing

A blood test that identifies a person's tissue type.

Toxins

Poisons. One of the main functions of the kidneys is to remove toxins from the blood.

Transplant

A term used to mean either a transplanted kidney (or other transplant organ) or a transplant operation.

Transplantation

The replacement of an organ in the body by another person's organ. Many different organs can now by successfully transplanted, including the kidneys, liver, bowel, heart, lungs, pancreas, skin and bones.

Transplant operation

The surgical operation by which a patient is given a donated organ. A transplanted kidney is placed lower in the abdomen than the patient's own kidneys, which are usually left in place.

Transplant waiting list

A list of patients awaiting transplantation, held locally or nationally. The national list is coordinated nationally by UKTSSA, whose computer compares patients' details (including blood group and tissue type) with those of cadaveric organs that become available.

Tunnel infection

Complication of peritoneal dialysis. It occurs when an infection spreads from the exit site into the 'tunnel' (ie the route of the PD catheter through the abdominal wall).

Ultrafiltration

The removal of excess water from the body. Ultrafiltration is one of the two main functions of the kidneys. In kidney failure, problems with ultrafiltration result in fluid overload. Dialysis provides an alternative means of ultrafiltration.

Ultrasound scan

A method of obtaining pictures of internal organs, such as the kidneys, or of an unborn baby, using sound waves. A device that sends out sound waves is held against the body. The sound waves produce echoes, which the scanner detects and builds up into pictures.

Urea

A waste product of protein breakdown normally removed by the kidney. When the kidney fails it accumulates in the bloodstream.

Ureters

The tubes that take urine from the kidneys to the bladder.

Urethra

The tube that takes urine from the bladder to the body surface.

Urinary catheter

A plastic tube inserted into the bladder for the removal of urine.

Urine

The liquid produced by the kidneys, consisting of the toxic waste products of food and the excess water from the blood.

Virus

A type of organism (much smaller than a bacterium) responsible for a range of mild and serious illnesses.

Vitamin D

A chemical that helps the body to absorb calcium from the diet. Blood levels of one form of vitamin D (calcitriol) are usually low in people with kidney failure.

Appendix D

Abbreviations

AAC	African or Afro-Caribbean
AAMI	Advancement of Medical Instrumentation
Ab	Antibody
ABLE	'A better life through education' (NKRF programme)
ACE	Angiotensin converting enzyme
ACDP	Advisory Committee on Dangerous Pathogens
Ag	Antigen
APD	Automated peritoneal dialysis.
ARF	Acute renal failure
AVF	Arterio venous fistula
BAPEN	British Association for Parenteral or Enteral Nutrition
BAPN	British Association of Paediatric Nephrology
BBV	Blood-borne virus
BMI	Body mass index
BP	Blood pressure
BS	British standard
BSA	Body surface area
CAPD	Continuous ambulatory peritoneal dialysis.
CANUSA	Canada or USA Collaboration Study
CCPD	Continuous cycler-assisted peritoneal dialysis
CENELEC	European Committee for Electrotechnical Standardisation
CFU	Colony forming units
CI	Confidence interval
CJD	Creutzfeld-Jakob disease
COPD	Chronic obstructive pulmonary disease
CMV	Abbreviation of cytomegalovirus.
CPA	Clinical pathology accreditation
CPD	Continuous peritoneal dialysis
CRF	Chronic renal failure
CRP	Chronic reactive protein
CVP	Central venous pressure
DCCT	Diabetes Control and Complications Trial
DOPPS	Dialysis Outcomes and Practice Patterns Study
DOQI	Dialysis Outcomes Quality Initiative
ECG	Electrocardiogram

ECHO	Echocardiogram
ELISA	Enzyme-linked innumosorbent assay
EPO	Erythropoietin (epoetin)
ES	European standard
ESRD	End-stage renal disease
FACS	Flucouresence activated cell sorter
FDA	Food and Drug Administration (US Department of Health and Human Services)
FDIS	Final draft international standard
GFR	Glomerular filtration rate
GP	General Practioner
HA	Health authority
HB	Health board
Hb	Haemoglobin
Hb AIC	Glycosylated haemoglobin
HBV	Hepatitis B virus
HCV	Hepatitis C virus
HD	Haemodialysis
HDF	Haemodiafiltration
HDL	High density lipoprotein
HDU	High dependency unit
HES	Hospital episode statistics
HIV	Human immunodeficiency virus
HLA	Human major histocompatibility complex
HMG-CoA	3 Hydroxy - 3 Methylglutaryl - Co- Enzyme A
HSP	Highly sensitised patient
Ht SDS	Height standard deviation scheme
HUS	Haemolytic uraemic syndrome
ICED	Index of co-existing disease
ICD	International classification of diseases
ICNARC	Intensive Care and National Audit and Research Centre
ICU	Intensive care unit
IDPN	Intradialytic parenteral nutrition
IEC	International Electrotechnical Commission
IPAA	Intra peritoneal amino acids
ISO	International Organisation for Standardisation
ISPD	International Society for Peritoneal Dialysis
iPTH	Immonoreactive parathyroid hormone
Kt/V	Measurement of dialysis adequacy
LAL	Limulus ameobocyte lysate

LDL	Low-density lipoprotein
LRD	Living-related donor
LRT	Living-related transplant
LVH	Left ventricular hypertrophy
LV	Left ventricle
MAG	Malnutrition Advisory Group
MDA	Medical Devices Agency
MDRD	Modification of diet in renal disease
MSBT	Microbiological safety of blood and tissues for transplantation
MW	Molecular weight
Mmol/l	Millimoles per litre. A unit used to measure the blood levels of many substances. Creatinine is measured in smaller units called micromoles per litre µmol/l.
MRSA	Methicillin resistant staphylococcus aureus
NAPRTCS	North American Paediatric Renal Transplant Study
NESP	Novel erythropoeisis stimulating protein
NFK – DOQI	National Kidney Foundation – Dialysis Outcome Quality Initiative
NG	Nasogastric
NIPD	Nocturnal intermittent peritoneal dialysis
NKRF	National Kidney Research Federation
PCR	Protein catabolic rate
PCT	Primary Care Trust
PD	Peritoneal dialysis
PEG	Percutaneous endoscopic gastrostomy
PET	Peritoneal equilibration test
PHLA	Public Health Laboratory Service
PICU	Paediatric intensive care unit
PNA	Protein nitrogen appearance
PRA	Panel reactivity antigen
prEN	provisional European standard
PTFE	Poly tetra
PTH	Parathyroid hormone.
RCT	Randomised control trial
rh GH	Recombinant human growth hormone
RNA	Ribo nucleic acid
RRF	Residual renal function
RRT	Renal replacement therapy
SA	Staphylococcus aureus
SGA	Subjective global assessment
SMR	Scottish Morbidity Record

SPA	Standard permeability analysis
TSAT	Transferrin saturation
UK-HARP	United Kingdom Heart and Renal Protection
UK-NEQAS	United Kingdom National External Quality Assurance Scheme
UKT	United Kingdom Transplant
UKTS	United Kingdom Transplant Service
UKTSSA	United Kingdom Transplant Support Service Authority.
ULTRA	Unrelated Live Transplantation Regulatory Authority. (This government body must give approval to all living unrelated transplants).
URR	Urea reduction rate
USRDS	United States Renal Database System
VRE	Vancomycin-resistant enterococcus
WHO	World Health Organisation
YORK CRD	Centre for Reviews and Dissemination
YORK DARE	Database of Abstracts of Reviews of Effectivenenss

Appendix E

Commercial affiliations of contributors

Chair

Alison M MacLeod Research project funded by Ortho Biotec (1999–2000). Travel expenses to meeting funded by Ortho Biotec and Fresenius.

Members /Authors

Mark T Bevan Lecture fees and travel expenses to conferences funded by Roche. Research support from Roche, Amgen and Ortho Biotec.

Gerald A Coles No commercial affiliations.

Andrew Davenport Travel expenses to meetings hosted by drug and dialysis companies. Research project funded by Fresenius.

Simon Davies Lecturing and consultancy work for Baxter (Advisory Board for CFPD, expert reports, research projects and research funding). Gambro (PD Advisory Board).

Terry Feest Lecture fees/Honoraria and/or conference expenses from Amgen, Astra Zeneca, Fresenius and Roche.

John Firth Has served on advisory boards or given lectures sponsored by Roche (1998), Pfizer (1999) and Astra Zeneca (2001).

Ram Gokal Consultancy for ML Pharmaceuticals. Research projects funded by Amgen & Baxter. Projects and Advisory group Ortho Biotech.

Timothy Goodship Consultancy for Amgen and Fresenius. Research project funded by Amgen.

Peter Gower No commercial affiliations.

Roger N Greenwood Lecture fees/Honoraria and/or conference expenses from Amgen, Roche, Baxter and Ortho Biotec.

Nicholas A Hoenich No consultancies. No lecture fees from pharmaceutical or dialyser producers. Research project funded by Gambro Renal R & D and administered by the University of Newcastle-upon-Tyne.

Anthony Nicholls Lecture fees from Baxter, Fresenius, Novartis and Smith Kline Beecham. Audit support from Ortho Biotec. Meeting support from Roche and Novartis.

Andrew J Rees No commercial affiliations.

Lesley Rees No commercial affiliations.

Paul Roderick Project part-funded by Baxter (1999–2000). Projects funded by Baxter (1999–2000), Pfizer (1998) and Roche (1998).

R Stuart C Rodger   Consultancy for Pfizer.

Alasdair Short   No commercial affiliations.

Charles RV Tomson   Lecture fees/Honoraria and/or conference expenses from Amgen, Astra, Baxter, Bayer, Fujisawa, Ortho Biotec, Novartis and Roche.

Robert Wilkinson   Lecture fees MSD, BMS, Sanofi, Pfizer, Bayer, Advisory Board MSD, BMS.

Adrian S Woolf   No commercial affiliations.